WHY DIE?

WHY DIE?

A Beginner's Guide to Living Forever

HERB BOWIE

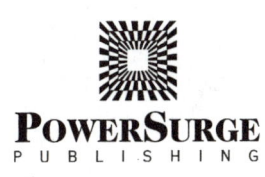

POWERSURGE
PUBLISHING

SCOTTSDALE, ARIZONA

Why Die?: A Beginner's Guide to Living Forever. Copyright © 1998 by Herb Bowie. All rights reserved, including the right of reproduction in whole or in part in any form. No part of this book may be reproduced or transmitted in any form or by any means, electronic or mechanical, including photocopying, recording, or by any information storage and retrieval system, without permission in writing from the publisher.

The ideas and suggestions in this book are not intended to replace the services of a trained health professional. It is recommended that the reader consult such a professional in matters relating to his or her health, and particularly in respect to any symptoms that may require diagnosis or medical attention. Any application of the recommendations set forth in the following pages is at the reader's discretion.

Throughout this book trademarked names are used. Rather than put a trademark symbol in every occurrence of a trademark name, we state we are using the names only in an editorial fashion and to the benefit of the trademark owner with no intention of infringement on the trademark.

Cover design by Foster & Foster, 1-800-472-3953. Printed and bound in the United States of America by Gilliland Printing.

To order additional copies of this book, or other products from PowerSurge Publishing, please see your favorite bookstore, or use the order form at the back of this book.

PowerSurge Publishing
PO Box 14707 • Scottsdale AZ 85267-4707 USA
1-602-451-6895 • Fax : 1-602-657-0727 • Toll-free: 1-800-925-3248
e-mail: info@www.powersurgepub.com
World Wide Web at http://www.powersurgepub.com

First printing: January 1998

1998 1999 2000 2001 2002 10 9 8 7 6 5 4 3 2 1

Library of Congress Catalog Card Number: 97-66499

Publisher's Cataloging-in-Publication
(Provided by Quality Books, Inc.)

Bowie, Herb.
    Why die? : a beginner's guide to living forever / Herb Bowie.
— 1st ed.
    p. cm.
    ISBN: 1-890457-07-8
    Includes bibliographical references and index.
    1. Immortalism. 2. Conduct of life. I. Title.
BF637.C5B68 1998   158.1
                    QBI97-40477

Dedication

To Pauline:

*Who made it clear,
from the very beginning,
that nothing less than forever
would do;*

and

To Charles Paul Brown,
Bernadeane Brown &
James Russell Strole:

*Three people whose lives and words
have transformed the idea of living
forever into a daily reality.*

Why die?

Because you think you have no other choice?

Because your ancestors did?

Because it's the "right thing" to do?

Instead …

Why not live?

Because you're **worthy to,**

Because you **want to,**

Because you're a **vital part** of the global human community.

Table of Contents

Preface ix

I. THE VISION 1
   1. Immortality in the 21st Century 3

II. BEGINNINGS 17
   2. My Kind of Immortality 19
   3. The Big "D" 27
   4. Allowing Uncertainty 31
   5. Turning Points 39
   6. Try Something New! 47

III. THE DECISION TO LIVE 51
   7. Determine Your Immortality Quotient 53
   8. Your Desire To Live 57
   9. The Benefits of Your Beliefs 71
   10. The Three Major Belief Systems 75
   11. Your Test Results Are Back 79

IV. HOW TO LIVE FOREVER 83
   12. The Fifteen Minimum Requirements 85

V. FEELINGS 97
   13. A Forever Kind of Feeling 99
   14. Embracing the Unknown 105

VI. SCIENCE 111
   15. Foundations 113
   16. Physics 117
   17. Biology 125
   18. Our Human Nature 137
   19. A Turning Point 147

VII. VALUE SYSTEMS 153
   20. Prioritizing Our Values 155
   21. Resolving Our Contradictions 161
   22. An American Tragedy.......................... 169

VIII. HUMAN RELATIONSHIPS 173
   23. Social Consequences 175
   24. A New Togetherness........................... 183
   25. Human Gravity – Falling Into One Another 191
   26. Social Structures 195
   27. Immortal Support Systems.................... 199
   28. Technology and the Human Web 203

IX. RELIGION 211
   29. Physical Immortality: The Un-Religion 213
   30. God 225
   31. The New Age 229

X. WHAT WE SEE IN THE MIRROR 239
   32. A New Self-Image 241

XI. APPLIED IMMORTALITY 249
   33. Immortal Parenting 251
   34. Rebirthing 259

XII. WHERE TO GO FROM HERE 263
   35. Immortality and You 265
   36. Seven Ways to Change the World 271
   37. Next Steps................................... 281

Notes 285
Recommended Reading 289
Index 295

Preface

IF YOU'VE ALWAYS BELIEVED that physical immortality is possible, but have been confused because there seemed to be no one else who felt that way – then this book is for you.

If you've already discovered others who feel that they too were born to live, and you now wish to deepen your feelings of living forever – then this book is also for you.

If you can't think of a good reason to go on living another year, or even another day – much less for all of eternity – then this book is for you as well. Living forever is all about transforming the quality of your life today, and these pages can help inspire that transformation.

And yes, even if you think that physical immortality is the craziest thing you've ever heard of – then this book is for you too. Because by the time we're done, you may just see why living forever is the most sensible thing you've ever started.

First Impressions

I chose the title of this book – "Why Die?" – because I knew it would be provocative. Many people make the unconscious decision that they have to die. They assume that their fate is ordained by the laws of nature, or the laws of God. This choice is made so early in life, and at such an unconscious level, that few people ever even challenge it. So I wanted to ask a question that would shake people up. Because even to ask this question is to imply something unthinkable for many people – that death is a choice, and not a foregone conclusion.

The book's subtitle – "A Beginner's Guide to Living Forever" – also deserves a bit of explaining. Many people feel disoriented and threatened by the consideration of physical immortality as a real possibility. I thought it might be comforting to have a guide that would lead the reader through such unfamiliar territory. The idea of a "Beginner's Guide" seemed particularly reassuring, although – to be honest – I don't think any other sort of book on this subject is possible. For no matter how long anyone may live, we will all and always be beginners when it comes to being here forever.

Forever and a Day

To understand the idea of living forever as I know it, we must look at two very different aspects of physical immortality. On the one hand, it is about eternity, about surviving to some unthinkably distant point in the future. On the other hand, though, it is all about choosing how to live our lives today. It is only when we connect these two extremes, and find a way to live our lives as an unbroken continuum between these two points, that we achieve what I call physical immortality.

This may seem like a paradox – to ask you to focus on forever and your life today at the same time. This is the way it first sounds when people show you what are called "Magic Eye" pictures, and tell you to focus beyond the page, on infinity. But if you relax and follow along, then after a while something new and different really does appear.

This paradox is also expressed in these haunting lines from William Blake.

> To see a world in a grain of sand
> And a heaven in a wild flower,
> Hold infinity in the palm of your hand,
> And eternity in an hour.

I am not speaking metaphorically though. In this book, I will be talking about transforming the quality of our lives today, by focusing our attention on our own eternity. At the same time, I will be talking about actually living for hundreds and thousands of years, by focusing our attention on the quality of our lives today. If this seems like a paradox, then this is only because we view our todays and our tomorrows as separate and unconnected.

Physical immortality is difficult, in a way, to talk about at length, because it can be approached from so many different angles. Since all of these perspectives are equally valid, it is impossible to do the subject justice by discussing it in a strictly linear fashion. We can start with forever and work backwards. We can start with today and go forwards. We can talk about the fate of humanity, or we can discuss the personal feelings of one individual. No matter how we approach the subject, though, we always seem to arrive at the same conclusion: that living forever is a practical and meaningful goal.

Reaching the same conclusion from so many different starting points is reassuring in the long run, but can be a bit disconcerting at first, as we repeatedly shift perspectives. You may feel more comfortable with some approaches than with others, and so may be tempted to skip around. The book will make the most sense, though, if you read it all from front to back.

The Path Ahead

I think you deserve a road map for the journey you are about to take, so let me give you some idea of the exciting trip that lies ahead.

Part I, "The Vision," offers a fictional look into the next century. This narrative focuses on one couple as they experience the possibility of living forever. The story gives a good overview of what I mean by physical immortality, and introduces many ideas that I will expand on later in the book.

Part II, "Beginnings," includes several different chapters that, in different ways, start our discussion of living forever. Our culture has produced many different images of physical immortality, so I'll tell you exactly what I mean by the term. I'll also talk about the origins of the idea, pointing out that the idea of living forever is not really as strange as it may first seem. You may be surprised to hear what some experts in related fields have to say on the subject. Finally, I will look at the case of someone who decided to stick with the safety of conventional beliefs, and strongly suggest that you try something different.

Part III, "The Decision to Live," suggests that life and death are the results of decisions we make, and not things that just happen to us. I'll give you a straightforward quiz that will determine your IQ (Immortality Quotient). Many forms of social conditioning prepare us to pack it in after only 70 or 80 years, and these will be pointed out. Also included here will be a discussion of the benefits that a belief in your own physical immortality can have on your life today.

Part IV, "How To Live Forever," reveals what I call the 15 minimum requirements for physical immortality. I believe that these techniques are bound to improve your life today, and offer real hope of extending our lives indefinitely.

Part V, "Feelings," talks about the importance of recognizing and nurturing our feelings of being here forever. In this part of the book I talk about what it feels like to look forward to eternity.

The next part of the book looks at the possibility of human physical immortality from a scientific perspective. I point out that the physical and biological sciences have found no fundamental principles that would make immortality impossible. I also explain why I think that the phenomenon of evolution has brought humankind to the brink of a new phase of history, in which immortality is our next logical step.

Human value systems are a subject of utmost importance to the survival of our race. In Part VII, I'll explain how the idea of physical immortality can help us transform and unify these values.

Life would be meaningless without other people in our lives. In Part VIII, I'll tackle the subject of "Human Relationships." We'll see how the decision to live forever can improve the quality of our connections to others, at a global as well as a personal level.

Almost all of us have been raised in one or more religious systems, and all of us have grown up in the shadow of religion. In Part IX, I'll explain how physical immortality is the next step in the evolution of religion.

Seeing ourselves as living forever has a profound impact on other aspects of our individual and collective self-images, and I talk about this in the next part of the book.

Part XI gives some examples of how the principles of living forever can be applied to other areas of life, such as parenting and bodywork.

In the last part of this book, I share with you some possibilities for further development of your immortality. You'll find some suggestions for what to do next, now that you have all eternity to look forward to!

Well, that's it – a brief tour of what's in store for you. I hope you find the possibilities as exciting as I do!

Part I

The Vision

Chapter 1. Immortality in the 21st Century

How would our world change if people stopped dying? I don't claim any special ability to foresee the future, but I thought it would be fun to start out with a vision of what our next 100 years might be like.

This first chapter offers a fictional look into the next century. The narrative focuses on one couple as they experience the possibility of living forever. This speculative look at possible developments in the 21st century presents a broad vision of what I mean by "living forever." Later in the book I will expand on many of the points I only touch on here.

Chapter 1

Immortality in the 21st Century

2002: Scientists Proclaim Immortality!

IN FEBRUARY, A GROUP OF SCIENTISTS shocked the world by announcing that, three years earlier, the human race had achieved a kind of theoretical immortality. It was at this point, they said, that the ever quickening pace of scientific discovery had reached a new and significant level. They had reached the point at which, for every year of additional research, at least one year could be added to the human life span. Although no guarantees could be made, there was little doubt that progress would continue at the same, if not a greater, rate. Eternity had arrived, then, not from a single "silver bullet," but from a snowball effect produced by the constantly increasing accumulation of relevant scientific advances.

Paul and Sara O'Connell were as astonished by the announcement as was the rest of the human race. Paul was an environmental engineer who had just turned 40, and his wife, originally from Israel, was a kindergarten teacher approaching her 37TH birthday. They and their seven year old son,

Stephen, had all spent their lives so far relatively free from accident and illness, and pursued life styles healthier than most. The "Immortality Proclamation," as it was called, caused Paul and Sara to stop and consider their options. Although neither of them seriously believed they could live forever, the possibility of extending their lives by a decade or two proved to be motivation enough. They began to seek out news of longevity research, and to apply it to their lives wherever possible.

2003: Humanity Faces the Choice to Live

Many other people were equally interested in the Proclamation. Scientific news that had previously been confined to technical journals or a few specialty magazines suddenly began appearing in most of the popular media. Newspapers began running columns on the subject of life extension, and many of these quickly grew into entire sections. Soon every major television network had at least two shows on the subject, and an entire cable channel devoted to longevity followed shortly thereafter.

Surprisingly, not everyone was excited with the possibility of living forever. As the number of people pursuing "incremental immortality" increased, so did active opposition to the movement. Since every major religion was based on some form of an afterlife, much antagonism came from this quarter. Even people who were not particularly religious seemed to feel that immortality was unnatural and somehow immoral. Others protested that dramatically lengthening human life spans invited some sort of apocalyptic catastrophe, such as mass starvation or economic collapse.

What followed was one of the most divisive social conflicts in history. For the first time, humanity was offered a clear choice between life and death. Science was outlining quite specific actions that could, when taken together, extend life spans dramatically. When faced with this option, many people declined. These same people, a few years ago, had shown no obvious signs of wanting to die. And yet, now that they had turned their backs on immortality, they seemed to court death with a vengeance. It soon became apparent that there was no middle ground in this division that crossed all existing socioeconomic and demographic categories. One was either a "lifer," as they came to be known, or one turned towards death.

Paul and Sara were troubled by religious and moral qualms from time to time, but had their new direction in life constantly reinforced by the improving quality of their lives. They not only expected to live longer in the future, they realized they felt better, and more alive, today. Of their parents, only Sara's mom was supportive of their decision, and even she did not choose to pursue life extension herself.

Paul changed jobs this year, at a significant decrease in salary, to get away from a boss who was adamantly anti-life. By the end of the year, Paul heard that his former boss had died of previously undiagnosed cancer. By this time, though, Paul was already firmly established at a new firm composed mostly of lifers, and there was no turning back.

2004: Immortality Groups Form

Paul and Sara joined a local immortality group that had formed recently. These started as study groups, distributing new information when it became available. They soon became support groups as well, with people helping each other to make the sometimes difficult changes in their lives that were demanded by the emerging longevity research.

2005: The Aliveness Meter

Much of the most promising research into human health was now taking place in the fields of psychology and sociology, as scientists further confirmed the importance of the body-mind connection. With these principles becoming more firmly established, immortality groups such as the one the O'Connells had joined became places to practice these principles, and not just to study them.

This field of inquiry was accelerated greatly by a discovery made by a physicist. Quite by accident, while searching for a new way to detect black holes, she discovered an entirely new form of radiation. It did not take her long to realize that the source of this energy was not a distant celestial body, but some quite close human bodies. She developed a meter with which to measure this field. Using this device, she found that the radiation was not constant, but fluctuated greatly from person to person, and from time to time with the same person. Interestingly, she discovered that it was often strongest with young people, and frequently weaker with older people.

She took some measurements in a variety of environments, including a hospital and a nursing home, where levels turned out to be particularly low. In the hospital she found one patient in particular whose output of this new energy field was barely perceptible. She made some discreet inquiries of the staff, without uncovering any reason for this unusual variation. When she arrived home, though, she found a message waiting for her that the patient had died from a sudden and quite unexpected heart failure.

Further and more methodical research confirmed that levels of this new radiation had a very high correlation with other measurements of health, including life expectancies for medical patients with critical conditions. Once this relationship was firmly established, the next step was to use this measuring device to find other factors that influenced the strength of this aliveness radiation, as it was now being called.

2006: Meter Validates Group in Arizona

Scientists from a number of different fields began to experiment with this new tool, but the most promising results were obtained by psychologists and sociologists. It turned out that the quality and quantity of human thought, feeling and interaction had a much more direct effect on the level of this new radiation than did any other factors.

One of the sociologists who had begun serious experimentation with the new "aliveness meter," as it had been dubbed by the popular press, was based at Arizona State University. He began to take readings at a variety of local religious services, with some varied and dramatic results. As he continued his research by investigating some religious organizations that were farther from the mainstream, he heard about a local group whose principles were actually based on human immortality. He attended one of their services, and was surprised to find that levels of aliveness radiation were off the scale of his meter.

He returned to his laboratory, calibrated the machine to ensure that there was nothing wrong with it, and then returned to the group's next meeting with a new machine, built to measure a higher range. This trip validated his earlier findings. He began to study the principles and practices of this organization, and soon published research that revolutionized the field of longevity.

The immortality groups that already existed turned out to be ideal forums to implement these new principles, and as a result they spread rapidly. Paul, Sara and Stephen adapted to them quickly, finding that they felt good, as well as being theoretically good for them. The idea of living forever was starting to sound appealing, as well as possible.

2009: A New Quality of Life

Some people had anticipated that the easing of the pressure of time would make people's lives less exciting. They worried that people who had "all the time in the world" would become so laid back that they might *appear* to be dead, even if they *were* going to live forever. It was true that people no longer felt the same pressure to cram a certain amount of achievement into a fixed number of years. It turned out, though, that research established a direct correlation between improving the quality of one's life today and increasing one's life expectancy. And since immortality had been granted, not through some magical fountain of youth or potion, but through people's own continuing and expanding efforts, people's general levels of involvement, commitment and excitement rose commensurately. Excitement, it turned out, was a prerequisite for immortality.

Paul and Sara were happier than they had ever been, but then they had by now been saying this for years. They both had lost weight, and looked younger and more fit than the day of the Proclamation seven years ago. They had become more involved in their careers, while at the same time keeping a balance with other aspects of their lives. Stephen would be going to college in four more years, but neither of them experienced any dread at being left alone in their house. They had experienced, through their weekly immortality meetings, a richness and a variety of human relationships that would allow them no thought of loss. They had other children that they were close to, as well as adults of all ages. Although they knew they would miss Stephen, they felt no threat of being emotionally deprived as he assumed a smaller role in their lives.

2014: Accidents On The Decline

The most persistent rub in the expanding possibility of immortality was the remaining threat from catastrophic accidents. No matter how healthy you became, people reasoned, it would do you little good if you were run over by a truck. When researchers finally turned their attention to this problem, they found that "accidents" were not as accidental as people had previously thought. People radiating higher levels of the aliveness radiation were found to be correspondingly less likely to have accidents. They also found that, as people became less resigned to eventual death, they were less tolerant of unsafe conditions that led to accidents in the first place. People were no longer satisfied with statistics that reported huge numbers of people dying each year in traffic accidents, for example. Accidental deaths were no longer just things to be watched on the evening news, they increasingly became invitations for positive action to make sure they didn't recur.

2021: Population Growth Stabilizes

People who had been worried about overpopulation by now realized that their fears had been misplaced. Although birth rates remained high in the diminishing number of relatively poor countries, they continued to decline in the richer countries, and especially among the lifers. These declining birth rates more than made up for the decrease in the death rates. It was not that these longer-lived people lost any interest in children – on the contrary, they seemed to enjoy them more than ever. At the same time, the immortality groups offered a new social structure that allowed fewer children to be enjoyed by more people, and allowed them to be shared across traditional family boundaries. These groups also relieved many of the former disadvantages of raising "only children," since these children now had other children within the groups that they could play with and become close to. These other children in the group replaced a few brothers or sisters with a larger number of "cousins."

The declining birth rates also seemed to be caused by other, more subtle, factors. The span of people's potential childbearing years continued to lengthen in parallel with their total life spans. This created even more of an environment in which having a child was a matter of choice, rather than a pre-programmed action triggered by a biological time clock. Also, as people's lives lengthened, and the prospect of living even longer became more real, they seemed less driven to achieve immortality through their offspring. Finally, the adult lifers were more childlike themselves, and seemed to rely less on the presence of children for that quality of joy so often associated with childhood.

Paul and Sara were no exceptions. They had adjusted to Stephen's adulthood and departure from their household. Although their doctors assured them that they could have another child if they wanted, they had never seriously considered it. They were still close to their son, and he delighted them as much now as he had in his first month.

Stephen, meanwhile, had married a girl he had met and fallen in love with in college, named Maggie. They were open to having a child, but were in no hurry, and felt no pressure from their parents, who already had plenty of contact with children of all ages. Stephen had become an aeronautical engineer, and Maggie was a journalist.

2027: Work Lives Change Dramatically

Widespread changes had taken place in people's working lives. Fears of a huge population of retired senior citizens utterly depleting their various pensions and retirement funds had proven ironically unfounded. Research, in fact, had confirmed many people's suspicions that retirement was inherently incompatible with radical life extension. With the siren song of retirement finally silenced, people were able to seriously turn their attention to improving working conditions. Employers granted more holidays and vacations each year, shortened the standard work week, and more frequently gave their employees paid sabbaticals from the workplace.

At the same time, as the principles of immortality became more widespread, people increasingly demanded that they be implemented in their working environments. The previous trend towards working at home and telecommuting reversed itself, as people started to look forward to going to work to be with other people there.

None of these advances were free, but society found ways to pay for them. As the span of productive working years increased, while the length of the expensive early years of life remained fixed, society found that its tax base was increasing while its education expenses were declining. Employees also became less fixated with constantly increasing salaries, as the need to accumulate a "nest egg" to finance the "golden years" of retirement became a diminishing reality. Retirement plans that had previously been funded by government agencies or employers either decreased their requirements or were liquidated altogether. Medical costs also declined, as more emphasis went into prevention rather than expensive and often ineffective correction. In general, the cost of living went down as people realized that most of their money had previously gone towards, not living, but bearing and raising children, getting sick and growing old.

Paul celebrated his 65TH birthday by liquidating his Individual Retirement Account, which by now held close to one million dollars, and using part of the money to start his own company. The new firm designed, manufactured and marketed recycling equipment. Sara went to work in the new company as well, and turned her educational skills towards training their customers in the use of the equipment. They found that working as well as living together enriched their relationship in new ways. Once again, they were happier than they had ever been.

2036: One Career No Longer Enough

Along with all the other changes in the workplace, "career hopping" was becoming more common. As more money and time became available for living, adults spent more of both on education. As life spans lengthened, it had become increasingly apparent that one dose of early education, no matter how big, would not be enough to last a lifetime – a program of ongoing "booster" shots would be necessary. Anyway, as people had become used to ongoing learning in the field of longevity, they began to extend their renewed interest in learning into other fields as well.

Some people built on earlier careers and knowledge bases to launch new ones. Others started with no more than a latent passion, and branched off in directions entirely different from ones previously taken. In either case, the decreased "cost of living" and modified retirement expectations allowed them to adjust joyfully to initially smaller salaries in their new vocations. Their lessened incomes were more than adequately balanced by the increased sense of freedom that came with the possibility of starting over, not one, but many times.

Paul and Sara continued to prosper in their company. Stephen had quit his engineering job, had come to work for his parents briefly, and then had started a new career as an actor. He had softened the blow to the family income, however, by waiting for a year during which his wife had to take her compulsory management rotation in the office. This stint earned her a 20% bonus. By the end of the year, when she returned to her normal duties, Stephen was performing regularly in the local community, although he was still making only about one third as much money as before.

2048: Global Environment Improves

The rate of scientific advance over the last few decades had quietly achieved an even greater acceleration than that of the last century. As more money became available, more of it was spent on scientific research. The diminished need to retrain a new generation of researchers every decade was also having its effect. Major breakthroughs were being routinely achieved by scientists in their sixties, seventies and eighties who had been able to build on the successes of their youth rather than seeing their powers diminish with age.

These technological advances were some of the factors contributing to a gradual turnaround of the environmental decline that had plagued the world since the beginning of the industrial revolution. A more immediate cause, though, was the increased motivation of the voting population to do something about these problems. The simple truth was that asking people to save the earth for future generations had never worked very well. Now that people were concerned with saving it for themselves, they focused on the issues at hand with an insistence that had previously been reserved for aging voters facing cuts to social security benefits.

Whatever the reasons, the United Nations in this year announced that, for the first time since they had begun tracking the relevant statistics, the earth's environment had actually *improved* over the past year. The hard work was not over, but the world had turned the corner.

Paul and Sara's company, in its own small way, was part of this turnaround. They had achieved substantial financial success, and were thrilled with the report from the UN. They decided to celebrate by taking a year off to travel the world, and turned the company over to a trusted employee to run in their absence.

2062: A New World Order

Scientists had firmly established that emotions of human suppression, prejudice and hostility were life-threatening for the subjects as well as the objects of these feelings. This realization had gradually replaced strong feelings of racism, nationalism and separatism with an expanding acceptance of all human beings as fellow citizens of the world. Organized religion, the other great divider of people, had fallen into decline without the need of much scientific intervention. It turned out that people who were increasingly unafraid of death had little need for the comfort of traditional religious beliefs.

At the same time, there were feelings of devotion, spirituality and reverence that were found to be greatly life-enhancing. The immortality groups that now covered the globe found, however, that they did not need a god or a sacred text to invoke these feelings. Haltingly at first, and then with increasing abandon, they had begun to apply these feelings to each other. As people found they could feel holy about themselves and other people, not just at these meetings but in their everyday lives, more and more people became converts to this new way of life. Immortality became the religion to end all religions.

With these age-old barriers to togetherness crumbling, national governments began to assume a more reasonable and restricted role in human affairs. The United Nations began to take on more of the functions formerly reserved for these national bodies. It was in this year that all the countries of the world turned their national defense systems over to the control of this world body, to be used for peacekeeping missions only.

2068: An International Language

In February the International Standards Organization released ISO 3364-18, which defined an international standard for the English language. This monumental document, including a dictionary and a book of grammar, was the culmination of a ten-year effort by a global committee. The intent was not only to standardize the language, but to simplify it by eliminating as many of its maddening inconsistencies as possible.

This new document satisfied the long-standing need for a truly international language. English had long ago become the de facto standard, but countries having another primary language had still bristled at the idea of acknowledging a foreign language as their own. Esperanto had been briefly touted as a neutral alternative, but since not even its most vocal advocates actually knew it, implementation had proved impractical.

The work of the International Standards Organization, then, accomplished two important objectives. First, it made the language easier to learn by cleaning up many of its irregular spellings and constructions. Second, and more importantly, it gave countries where English was not the standard a chance to take ownership of the language by making changes to it.

In November, the United Nations adopted International English as its official language. Predictably, the strongest objections came from England, which was still having difficulty reconciling itself to the way America had bastardized the language. The eloquent objections of the language's mother country were overridden, though, and one more barrier to global communication was removed.

2090: Together Forever

One of the dire recurring predictions made by those skeptical of immortality was that human relationships could never last that long. These cynics insisted that those who had eagerly pledged to remain faithful until death did them part would all too quickly renounce their vows when staring into the face of eternity.

Although the conquest of all sexually transmitted diseases had given a certain impetus to this argument, many couples persisted despite the predictions. It was not that they were unattractive, or unattracted, to others. They enjoyed these erotic feelings without feeling any compelling need to consummate them, and these emotions became just one more strand in the rich and satisfying tapestry of their social existence.

Paul and Sara were one of many such fortunate couples. They celebrated their hundredth wedding anniversary by visiting a new resort on the moon. They looked back over their years together: time during which they had grown closer than they had ever thought possible, had shared and stimulated each other's growth, and had become people they had never dreamed of being when they were married. They drank a toast to each other, and pledged their love for the next hundred years, and made love together, for perhaps the ten thousandth time, as the earth sank beneath the horizon.

Part II

Beginnings

This section includes several chapters that, in different ways, start our discussion of living forever.

Chapter 2. My Kind of Immortality

Our culture has produced many different images of physical immortality, so I'll tell you exactly what I mean by the term.

Chapter 3. The Big "D"

Here I talk briefly about the only alternative to immortality, why it's necessary to talk about it, and the discomfort the subject causes

Chapter 4. Allowing Uncertainty

Most people feel certain that they will die someday. This chapter points out that the idea of living forever is not really as strange as it may seem at first. You may be surprised to hear what some experts in related fields have to say on the subject.

Chapter 5. Turning Points

Here I describe some of the influences in my own life that led me to embrace the reality of human physical immortality.

Chapter 6. Try Something New!

Finally, I look at the case of someone who decided to stick with the safety of conventional beliefs. I strongly suggest that you try something different.

Chapter 2

My Kind of Immortality

THE IDEA OF PHYSICAL IMMORTALITY conjures up many strange images in people's minds. I want to let you know exactly what I mean by the phrase. It's probably easiest to start through a process of elimination. There are many common notions that have little to do with what I am talking about.

No Spooks

I am not talking about any form of spiritual immortality. By "physical immortality," I don't mean anything having to do with an afterlife, angels, ascension, heaven or reincarnation. I'm not talking about a life after death, but about a life without death!

Neither am I discussing mysterious non-human life forms, whether they are extraterrestrials, the lost citizens of Atlantis, or strange underground civilizations.

Not An Elixir

Storytellers have often depicted physical immortality as achievable through some dramatic, irreversible action. Magic potions are popular. The vampire myth is an example of this, as are stories of zombies who come back from the grave and can no longer be killed: "the undead," as they are sometimes called. Taken as a group, this sort is generally not an attractive lot.

The 1992 film *Death Becomes Her*, directed by Robert Zemeckis and starring Meryl Streep, is a recent example of the type. This movie portrayed immortality as a state in which people could not die, even when their bodies were subject to injuries that would kill ordinary people.

I won't try to sell you on something that is the subject of myths and fables. I'm not talking about some magical state in which death is no longer possible. I'm talking about a decision to choose life instead of death.

More Than Longevity

Many experts today make recommendations about how to slow or stop the aging process. Some prescribe certain techniques to be followed, such as breathing techniques or particular forms of exercise. Many promote strict dietary guidelines. Others recommend vitamin, mineral, herbal or hormonal supplements to your diet.

Much of this advice is valuable. Yet there is a subtle paradox in many of these messages. Popular books have spoken of the ability to stop aging, to become ageless, or to remain youthful. Yet the same books (somewhere in the fine print) always claim that you still have to die someday. Some even disparage the idea of immortality, as if it were somehow sacrilegious, or anti-social.

These sorts of pundits have produced a curious new model

of human development. The healthy, affluent, intelligent person, by following their recommendations, is supposed to remain youthful, vibrant and sexy, right up to the moment at which they ... drop dead. The end result, one can only suppose, is a youthful corpse.

But what kills these robust, youthful figures? If not aging, then what? There seems to be an obvious contradiction here, even though most people's conditioning causes them to accept it without question.

Much of this anti-aging advice is valuable. It is also readily available from many different sources. I am not going to offer you anything new in this area. What I am going to do, though, is provide a new context for longevity, one that is worthy of the techniques that are becoming so plentiful today.

Not Just More of the Same

People often see physical immortality as nothing more than an indefinite extension of the life they have always had. Predictably, their reaction is usually, "Who needs it?"

I won't try to persuade you to merely prolong your existing life. I want to talk to you about achieving a whole new quality of living.

Physical immortality means more to me than just the ability to end the limitation of death: it represents, for me, the lifting of all arbitrary constraints on human development – for myself, for others I know, and for us as a species. To accept physical immortality is to accept the infinite possibilities of human existence. To accept the inevitability of death, on the other hand, is to acquiesce in the artificial limitations imposed by social and genetic programming. If I believe in living forever, then I believe in always having more. If I believe in a finite number of years, then I believe that what I have now is enough. For me, this difference in attitude has a far-reaching effect on all aspects of my life.

Something New

Although I think figures from our past have felt the desire for immortality, and have tried to live it, I do not believe that any have achieved it. I'm not going to be telling you about ancient secrets that have only recently been rediscovered. I won't hint at shadowy figures who have been living in the Himalayas for the past thousand years. I'm describing a new step for humanity, not something that has gone before.

Because I am talking about something new, there is a tendency to dismiss these ideas as preposterous. Remember, though, that there was a time when people laughed at the notion that the world was round. Everyone "knew" that it was flat, because that was the way it seemed. Yet today the situation has been reversed, and it seems absurd to suppose that the earth is flat. There was a time when people laughed at the notion of human flight, saying that if we were meant to fly, God would have given us wings. And yet, the Wright Brothers flew. There was a time when people thought that it was impossible for a person to run a mile in less than four minutes. Yet, once Roger Bannister broke this barrier, many others soon achieved the same "impossible" feat.

So just because physical immortality hasn't happened yet, don't make the mistake of thinking that it isn't happening now.

A New Paradigm

For me, physical immortality is a new way of looking at the world, and at my part in it. It offers a fresh perspective on the universe. It is a radically new way of seeing.

If these seem like empty words, then think for a minute of the huge impact Christianity has had on human existence over the last 2,000 years. An impact produced by the recorded words of a single person with a new vision of what it meant to be human. And if you feel that it is sacrilegious to speak of improvements on Christianity, then recall for a moment the words of Christ himself:

> Verily, verily, I say unto you, He that believeth on me, the works that I do shall he do also; and greater works than these shall he do; because I go unto my Father.[3]

Human knowledge is usually acquired in an evolutionary fashion. One person builds on the work of another, and of others before him. New wisdom is carefully laid down one layer at a time, building on the foundations that have already been established.

Every so often, though, something different happens. A revolution occurs. An individual discovers a new way to look at the available data. This new way of organizing our knowledge is often simpler than the old way. It sheds new light on old wisdom, and explains things that remained mysterious within the old structures.

A good example of such a profound change in the structure of scientific belief was Einstein's theory of general relativity. Within the limits of most preceding experimental observations, Einstein's theory predicted results identical to those of previous theories. Outside of those normal limits, though, the new theory predicted such strange behavior as the slowing of time at speeds approaching that of light. Experimental confirmation subsequently proved Einstein's theory to be correct.

Thomas Kuhn, in his hugely influential book, *The Structure of Scientific Revolutions,* called these transformational experiences "paradigm shifts." Lately the use of this phrase has been extended to fields of human inquiry other than science.

The acceptance of immortality as a legitimate human goal requires just such a paradigm shift. It offers a new way of looking at human experience. It does not change the data that humanity has recorded up to this point. But, like Einstein's theory of general relativity, this new way of looking at things simplifies, combines and extends older perspectives, and points the way to new possibilities never before imagined.

You may have seen the following puzzle before. It is popular in courses on creativity.

> **Puzzle:** Connect all nine dots below, using only four lines, without retracing over any lines, and without lifting your pen or pencil from the paper.

•   •   •

•   •   •

•   •   •

Give up? If you had difficulty coming up with a solution, then it was probably because you assumed a constraint not actually stated in the problem. You probably tried to think of a solution that would stay within the "box" marked by the outside dots. The actual solution is as follows.

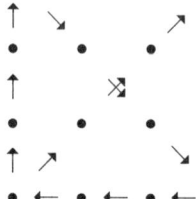

Start here

My Kind of Immortality

This puzzle provides a good illustration of how a different perspective can provide fresh solutions. As long as you keep thinking "inside the box," a solution is not possible. It is only when you start thinking "outside the box" that an answer becomes apparent.

Death is like the box in this puzzle. As long as people keep creating their lives "inside the box" of death, they will keep coming up with approaches that do not work completely. But when we take a fresh perspective, we can allow ourselves to think of what is possible once we allow ourselves to wander "outside the box." Only then we can take a new approach to life, and come up with fresh solutions. Once we set our sights on forever, we begin to see old problems in a new light.

Physical immortality offers humanity nothing less than a new consciousness. A consciousness, I believe, that will take us into the coming millennium and beyond. A consciousness that will radically transform the quality of human existence on this planet.

This radically new consciousness, this revolution in our way of thinking, is the subject of this book.

Chapter 3

The Big "D"

> Do not go gentle into that good night.
> Rage, rage against the dying of the light.[4]
>
> — Dylan Thomas

> We may all concede that we are going to die, but except in moments when we have to be present with the dead or dying, our dread is kept under wraps. This is almost a biological necessity – I can't imagine how I could keep going if the thought of my own death came to the surface of thought more than once or twice a year.[5]
>
> — Deepak Chopra

> It's not that I'm afraid to die. I just don't want to be there when it happens.[6]
>
> — Woody Allen

Fear

ONE OF THE BIGGEST BARRIERS to a serious consideration of physical immortality is our discomfort with thoughts of the only other alternative: death. Unfortunately, it is impossible to talk about the one without also mentioning the other.

Many people grow uncomfortable when physical immortality is discussed, because, consciously or subconsciously, the subject inevitably brings with it thoughts of dying.

As Chopra admits above, with characteristic insight and honesty, most people have a terrible fear of their own demise. They have grown expert, though, at keeping this dread under wraps. This is why surveys often show that people claim to be more afraid of public speaking than of death. It is not really that people find public speaking to be more terrible, but rather that people are not as well trained at suppressing their feelings about it!

The quotation from Woody Allen is also revealing. It is funny because it is so ridiculous, and yet at the same time so true. Most people claim that they are not afraid to die, but only because they never really see themselves as being there when it happens. They never fully allow themselves to feel the horror of death, and so they convince themselves that they are not frightened by it.

American society certainly helps people deal with their fear of death by ritualizing our approach to it. All feelings concerning death are carefully channeled into well established and rigidly defined behaviors. We prepare for our own deaths by buying life insurance and preparing our last will and testament. We deal with the deaths of others through funerals and religious ceremonies. We substitute for any real contemplation of death our traditional religious beliefs in an afterlife. Instead of letting ourselves get in touch with our true feelings, we quickly turn to these various rituals as more comfortable alternatives.

Paradoxically, our media's obsession with death and violence is really another symptom of this deep suppression. It seems impossible to go to the movies these days, or read a best selling book, or turn on prime-time TV, or read a daily newspaper, without being subjected to graphic carnage. The effects of this daily bombardment are twofold. The first result is to simply make us numb. We are subjected to images of death so often that we eventually stop reacting to these ritualistic stimulants.

The second effect of this media barrage is more subtle. The deaths depicted by the media are almost always sensational ones: bizarre accidents, psychotic killings, or criminal acts. What is rarely covered by the media are the routine deaths, the ones that happen under "normal" circumstances. The subliminal message seems to be that, if everyone were only normal like us, then none of this nasty stuff would happen. The result is that we are conditioned to think of death as a media event, rather than something that routinely happens to real people. We are encouraged to think of death as a series of isolated exceptions, and almost never invited to think about death as a general phenomenon.

A Secret Pact

There is something more at work, though. More than just a simple fear, people have a deep discomfort about frank and open discussion of death. This is because most people have made two unconscious agreements on the subject. The first is that people have agreed to die. The second agreement is to not discuss the first one.

You might think that death requires no agreement. The lines from Dylan Thomas remind us, though, that we have some choice in the matter. At the very least, we do not have to "go gentle into that good night." Instead, we can "Rage, rage against the dying of the light."

Most of us, though, have agreed to accept death. And we

have further agreed to go along with it quietly, by not even discussing this agreement. We have made a secret pact with the enemy. No wonder we grow uncomfortable when someone brings up the subject! To discuss immortality, though, we obviously have to bring this clandestine agreement out in the open, and look at it with eyes wide open.

Open Discussion

Some people accuse speakers on immortality of having a morbid desire to talk about death. I assure you that this is not the case, and that most of this book will be devoted to the subject of life. No discussion of this topic would be complete, though, without serious consideration of death as a phenomenon, and of our attitudes towards it. So I ask for your patience and your tolerance as we open up these subjects. At the same time, I invite you to become more whole by letting yourself fully experience your deepest feelings about life and death.

Chapter 4

Allowing Uncertainty

Death and Taxes

WHEN IT COMES TO THE SUBJECT OF DEATH, most Americans consider Benjamin Franklin to have been the ultimate authority. It was he who said, in 1789, "But in this world nothing can be said to be certain, except death and taxes."[7] For most people, this aphorism neatly sums up the common view of death: "Everyone has to die. There's nothing we can do about it. Let's forget about it and talk about things we can do something about."

But is death really such a sure thing? If you base your opinion on human experience thus far, then it's hard to draw any other conclusion. Even the most optimistic among us must admit that people have been dying with heartbreaking regularity for a very long time. So, if you believe that things will always be pretty much the same way they've always been, then you will clearly believe pretty strongly in the certainty of death.

Similar reasoning, however, has proven wrong in the past. Most people were once sure that the sun revolves around the earth. We now understand that it is our planet that orbits around the sun. Some once thought it impossible for human beings to travel faster than the speed of sound. But the sound barrier was nonetheless broken. There was a time when people laughed at the notion of space travel. Yet Neil Armstrong set foot on the moon, making a reality of what had previously been called science fiction. Of course, all these examples of "common sense" seemed sensible enough at the time. Is it possible that a belief in the certainty of death could also be wrong – perhaps dead wrong?

A Different Perspective

I happen to believe in the possibility of human physical immortality. I would like you to acknowledge this possibility as well. It's not just that I like people to agree with me. I think that this fundamental paradigm shift can cause a profound and wonderful change in the quality of human life on this planet. I think that this radical change in our perspective can help us create heaven on earth together. Before you can admit the possibility of living forever, though, you must let go of your certainty of death.

You may believe that this sounds crazy. You may believe that death is "natural." You may think that there is universal agreement on the inevitability of death. Many people share these mistaken beliefs. If I try to tell you that you're wrong, you'll likely discount what I have to say. So let me instead share with you some words from other people, from some acknowledged experts in their fields. I don't expect their words to convince you that you're going to live forever. But perhaps they can at least begin to open your mind to the possibility.

Science

Many people think that there are well-understood scientific principles that determine our fate. Everything breaks down eventually, they say. They see their car wear out, they see living organisms aging, and they mistakenly ascribe both phenomena to the same scientific law.

Such is not the case. The laws of physics do dictate that all closed systems will eventually deteriorate, gradually becoming less organized and more chaotic. But living beings are not closed systems, and are therefore not subject to what is known as the second law of thermodynamics. If we were, then we could not grow and mature, and we could not repair ourselves when we suffer injuries.

But are there biological laws that demand our ultimate demise? If there are, then the best scientists of our day have failed to discover them. Don't take my word for it, though. Listen to what they have to say.

> It is not obvious why aging should occur.[8]
>
> — Leonard Hayflick, Ph.D.

More than just not obvious, the reasons for aging turn out to be completely missing, as Hayflick finally admits later in the same volume.

> We know of no good reason why aging should happen.[9]
>
> — Leonard Hayflick, Ph.D.

Two other professors, in a different text, state much the same views in a more positive vein.

> Next to the miracle of life itself, aging and death are perhaps the greatest mysteries.[10]
>
> — Robert E. Ricklefs and Caleb E. Finch

Despite popular conceptions to the contrary, our best biologists and gerontologists frankly admit that they do not understand why we age and die.

So, if you have thought that you must die because science has discovered good reasons why it must be so, then you'll have to find some better reasons.

Ancient Spiritual Leaders

Other sources of people's confusion about death are their spiritual teachings. Almost all organized religions offer some sort of afterlife as solace for the necessity of physical death. Most forms of modern Christianity, for example, talk about eternal life only as a heavenly existence. Many people are surprised, then, to find that the Bible speaks openly of physical immortality.

> Yea, his soul draweth near unto the grave, and his life to the destroyers.
>
> If there be a messenger with him, an interpreter, one among a thousand, to shew unto man his uprightness.
>
> Then he is gracious unto him, and saith: Deliver him from going down to the pit: I have found a ransom.
>
> His flesh shall be fresher than a child's: he shall return to the days of his youth.[11]
>
> — Job 33:22–25

Many Biblical references to eternal life are often interpreted in a spiritual context, but this is clearly and dramatically physical. Life is spoken of as being destroyed by death. Death itself is referred to as "going down to the pit." And the alternative is depicted in unmistakably biological terms: "His flesh shall be fresher than a child's: he shall return to the days of his youth."

Following is another, simpler, reference.

> The last enemy that shall be destroyed is death.[12]
>
> — 1 Corinthians 15:26

Here, death is referred to, not as an entrance to some heavenly existence, but as an "enemy," to be "destroyed."

Following is one of the many references by Christ to physical immortality.

> Verily, verily, I say unto you, If a man keep my saying, he shall never see death.
>
> Then said the leaders unto him, Now we know that thou hast a devil. Abraham is dead, and the prophets; and thou sayest, If a man keep my saying, he shall never taste of death.
>
> Art thou greater than our father Abraham, which is dead? and the prophets are dead: whom makest thou thyself?[13]
>
> — John 8:51–53

> Jesus said unto them, Verily, verily, I say unto you, Before Abraham was, I am.[14]
>
> — John 8:58

This reference is perhaps the most unquestionably physical of all of Christ's comments on the subject. It begins with Jesus asserting that his followers will "never see death." (Note that he doesn't say that they will survive death, as he might if he was speaking of an afterlife – he says that they will never even see it.) The leaders respond as many current Christian leaders might, by saying that other, supposedly greater, figures have died before him – who does he think he is, anyway?

Christ's answer is simple, and it is interesting to note some of the things that he does *not* say. He doesn't say that Abraham and the prophets are all alive and well in heaven. He doesn't say that they will all rise from the dead together at some appointed future time. He doesn't disagree at all with the leaders' interpretation of Christ's statement as referring to physical life and death. He simply says, "Before Abraham was, I am."

Listen to what is being said here. Jesus says that his followers will experience endless life. An authority figure questions his statement. And Jesus doesn't at all back down, or explain away his claim. He simply asserts his authority to say such a thing.

Modern religious authorities may try to explain these statements away by way of various interpretations based on their own dogma. But a simple, unbiased reading of the text indicates clearly that the Bible is speaking of physical immortality as a desired and promised goal.

So, if you've been thinking that death is inevitable because it is part of the law of God, then you'll have to look elsewhere for justification.

Modern Spiritual Leaders

Many new spiritual movements also focus on reincarnation or some sort of afterlife as consolation for having to die. Yet the best of these also make statements alluding to the possibility and importance of living forever.

Deepak Chopra is one of the most popular of the New Age authors. His book, *Ageless Body, Timeless Mind* was a huge bestseller. In it, he quoted Shankara, one of the greatest of the Indian sages.

> "People grow old and die because they see others grow old and die."[15]
>
> — Deepak Chopra

This clearly indicates a belief that aging and death are results of conditioning and habit, rather than necessity.

Even more telling, I think, is this next passage. One of the great myths of many religions is the belief that spirituality is at odds with our physical existence. People speak of the body as being a disposable container for an immortal soul. Here, Chopra gives the lie to this common error.

> Spirituality is not meant to be separate from the body. Sickness and aging represent the body's inability to reach its natural goal, which is to join the mind in perfection and fulfillment. At every stage of spiritual growth, the greatest ally you have is your body.[16]
>
> — Deepak Chopra

Think of this: "At *every* stage of spiritual growth, the greatest ally you have is your body." So what does this say about death? If death represents a separation of spirit from body, then it can't be good for the spirit. On the contrary, physical immortality would seem to offer the greatest avenue of spiritual advancement.

So, if you think that New Age teaching gives you good reason for wanting to leave your body behind, then you might have to think again.

The Possibility of Physical Immortality

Most people go through life with the certainty of their own demise hanging over their heads like the sword of Damocles – they don't know exactly when it will fall, but they never doubt that one day it will.

What would it mean to live free from the sentence of death? And if it would mean a different life, then who has the power to lift this sentence, to start us on the path of this new existence?

Perhaps we hold this power in our own hands, in our own minds. And perhaps we can unleash it just by letting go of this iron grip that most of us have on the certainty of death. For once we acknowledge that death is uncertain, then immortality is more than just possible – it begins today.

Chapter 5

Turning Points

FOR THE LAST TEN YEARS, I have held the belief that people can and should live forever. What's more, I have associated with others who hold the same belief. We also believe that one of the keys to achieving this state of physical immortality is a new quality of human togetherness.

Many of my family members, friends and associates have a hard time understanding what has gotten into me. For most people, this idea of physical immortality, and this emphasis on togetherness, are difficult to relate to. These new beliefs and priorities appear to have come out of the blue. One day (they seem to think), Herb was walking around like any other person, normal to all outward appearances. Then – Bam! – suddenly he thinks he is immortal, and is consorting with this odd group of people. What happened?

For me, this is not at all how it looks. I was not subject to a sudden and unexpected conversion. Instead, I see my interest in physical immortality as the natural culmination of a long series of turning points, each one taking me a step closer to these people, to this life. Others have come by different routes, so there is no magic to these particular events. Yet all the experiences I describe here have been shared by many others. So perhaps by describing them, and what they have meant to me, it will be easier for others to come along, or at least to understand how I got here.

Religion

My parents tried. They really did. They raised me as a good Methodist. My faith in an omnipotent deity expired, though, one fateful spring after I discovered the box my chocolate egg had come in. In a flash, the awful truth dawned on me that the Easter bunny was a hoax.

By comparison, it was relatively easy to give up God. The story of the Easter bunny was at least a simple tale, even if untrue. The vast maze of Christian religious beliefs, in contrast, always held a note of artifice for me. I have generally found the truth to be relatively simple – unexpected, perhaps, but still convincingly simple. Religion, though, always sounded to me like a lie that had gone on for too long.

You know the kind. When you try to cover up the truth, you start by telling a simple lie. But then, if someone begins questioning you, trying to reconcile your lie with what they know to be true, you end up weaving an increasingly complex tapestry of falsehood. You pile one fabrication on top of another, until finally the whole structure seems tenuous and unstable. These types of stories, even when they successfully avoid any obvious contradictions, never quite seem convincing. Like bad scientific theories, they seem to introduce more questionable suppositions than they purport to explain. Even though they cannot be proven wrong, they lack the ring of truth.

Religion raised many important questions for me. Why are we here? How were we created? Why do people die? Yet the answers always struck me as too complicated to be true. None of the answers ever seemed to satisfy.

The Beatles

Like millions of other kids, I worshipped The Beatles. Their music, though, only partially explained their appeal to me. There was something else about them that seemed revolutionary, some trait always implied but never openly stated.

The Beatles had a togetherness that I longed for. Not the homogenized, uniform sameness that I saw around me, but something new, something that celebrated diversity and unity at the same time.

In the early years of their success, the fab four all dressed alike, all sported the same haircuts, all made the same music together. Yet they were not faceless band members. They all had distinct and obviously different personalities. And there was not a single front man, as in so many other groups. No one was in the foreground or background. Unlike any musical group before or since, they were often introduced on the radio simply by their first names: John, Paul, George and Ringo. More than just popular musicians, they seemed to be:

- four distinct individuals who at the same time formed a cohesive whole;

- people who came together for a common purpose without sacrificing their individuality;

- human beings who changed the world by forming a bond that went beyond conventional relationships of family, friends and work;

- people who transformed those around them, not through the words they spoke, but through the music they played, the jokes they made, their appearance, their very presence.

Catch-22

Joseph Heller's darkly comic novel had the ring of truth about it. It poked fun at the absurdity of religious beliefs, yet betrayed a deeply felt respect for the human ideals and longings embodied in these beliefs.

At the most literal level, *Catch-22* was about World War II. At a deeper level, it was about the absurdity of all war. At many points, though, Heller uses WWII as a metaphor for modern society in general, extending the reach of the book beyond the trenches of combat.

At its most basic level, though, this book speaks to a universal human condition. There are many "catches" in the book, many ways in which the characters are caught between hope and reality, between desire and possibility. Many of these catches seem pointless, the arbitrary decisions of a mindless bureaucracy. As the book progresses, though, and its central mystery is revealed, the ultimate "catch" becomes clear: we want to live, but we have to die. As Yossarian feels by the end of the book, there has to be a better way.

College

In 1969 I left my family home in Annapolis, Maryland and began four years of college at the University of Michigan, in Ann Arbor.

College was a magical place for me. It was like a storybook land. Sandwiched between the stark constraints of growing up with my family (as wonderful as they were), and the routine and responsibility of the working world, were four years of magnificent freedom.

I lived in a dormitory, and then apartment buildings, with other roommates. The confining expectations of families and bosses were nowhere to be found. I lived in a society whose purpose was learning and discovery of new truths: both in and out of the classroom, on and off campus. The traditional relationships of family members and coworkers were missing. I had friends. Beyond friendship, though, there was this tremendous sense of a common experience. It was an experience shared with the hundred or so students I met in classrooms each semester, the thousands I shared a campus with, and the millions in other colleges across the US, and around the world. We were being birthed by, and at the same time giving birth to, a new culture. I started in the school of Engineering, switched to Physics for a semester, then surrendered a scholarship so that I could major in English literature – for no better reason than that I felt drawn to it.

I have never lost this desire to be a co-creator of an emerging culture, to live in a society dedicated to learning and the discovery of new truths, new thoughts, and new realities.

The Films of Frank Capra

Among the many benefits of life in Ann Arbor were the various student film societies that screened recent and classic movies on a regular basis. If you wanted to, you could see a different film practically every night of the week. European films were all the rage on college campuses at this point, and many were darkly lit and full of despair.

One weeknight, in the middle of winter, I can remember going to a small auditorium with one of my best friends to see an old black-and-white American comedy. The director had been one of the most commercially successful of his generation. His films were currently out of style with academia, though, considered too sentimental and naively optimistic – full of "Capra corn," as they called it.

We sat in the dark for an hour and a half, surrounded by no more than a handful of fellow students. When the movie was over, we discovered it was snowing outside. We lived in different directions, and it was too late to go anywhere else, so we stood there in the deepening cold and falling snow and talked about the film we had just seen. We were so excited that we stayed there, talking in the dark, for what seems like at least an hour, before we could bear to go our separate ways.

The film was *You Can't Take It With You*, directed by Frank Capra, one of the acknowledged masters of the American cinema (his work has since come back into popularity). Other Capra films are *It Happened One Night, Meet John Doe, Mr. Smith Goes to Washington* and *It's A Wonderful Life*.

Viewed today, generally on television, squeezed between reruns of old sitcoms, it is easy to mistake Capra's films for trite Americana. Watch closely, though, and you will find deeply felt beliefs in the redemptive power of community and the ultimate sanity of quirky individuality, and an abiding mistrust of politics, big business and the media.

Capra's faith in the ultimate goodness of humanity was rocked by the same World War that gave birth to *Catch-22*. His films stirred in me a renewed hunger for this strange mix of togetherness and diversity.

Group Therapy

After college I moved to Los Angeles. Despite the handicap of having a degree in English, I stumbled across a job in computers, and found a career that was both interesting and financially rewarding.

I was not happy, though. My life felt empty. I had a few close friends, but nothing that really stirred me, really motivated me. A friend referred me to a therapist she had been seeing, a wonderful woman named Jennifer Reese. Jenny practiced Gestalt therapy, and after a few individual sessions she asked me to join one of her ongoing groups.

In society's eyes, the goal of therapy was to restore me to normality. In reality, though, group therapy opened up a whole new world for me. I found a level of emotional honesty that I had never before experienced. I found a setting in which people shared what was really going on within them, beneath the normal facades that got them through the day. I experienced a new sense of family, among the six to eight people in my group, and others I met at encounter weekends. People in Jenny's practice came from all walks of life, and all sorts of backgrounds. I felt nourished by this close communion with a group of people I never would have chosen, had I been left to choose on my own. I flourished in an atmosphere that encouraged personal growth and transformation, and not just dependable reliability.

In society's eyes, therapy was supposed to fix me and send my on my way. In reality, though, these few hours a week rekindled a hunger in me for a different way of life. I found what I had been missing, but it was only partially something that had been missing in me – it was also something missing from my daily life, and from the lives of those around me.

Marriage

In 1978 I met a wonderful woman with whom I seemed to have nothing in common. On our first date we attended a movie that I loved and that she hated. There was something that drew us together, though, despite our differences. Two years later we were married (with Jenny, my therapist, performing the ceremony). Nothing was said about "until death do us part." And inside the wedding band that Pauline gave me was a simple inscription: "Forever."

The Rebirthing Community

Through a friend, Pauline discovered a weekend seminar called the LRT – the Loving Relationships Training. The event included a group rebirth on Saturday evening. Rebirthing is a breathing technique that releases deep emotional memories, even allowing the breather to re-experience, and then release, the pain of their birth.

Much of what was taught on these weekends would now loosely be called part of "New Age" thinking. The LRT weekend encouraged people to take 100% responsibility for what happens to them. It included a section on physical immortality. The trainers encouraged people to see everything that happens as a choice, up to and even including death. And so, if we can choose death, then why not choose life instead?

Pauline and I attended many of these weekends, eventually becoming assistants ourselves. These were wonderful experiences, but we were finally left hungry for more. We enjoyed the community. We were eventually frustrated, though, because the community did not seem to be a primary goal, but an accidental byproduct of another process that was supposed to transform people and then send them on their way.

People Forever

In 1986 we moved to Arizona, and stumbled across a group called People Forever. Here, finally, we found what we had been looking for. Instead of the confusion of religion, we found a simple truth: people deserve to live. We found people who celebrated diversity and the uniqueness of each individual, yet who also wanted to build a togetherness strong enough to keep us together forever. We found an ongoing community of people who encouraged unending growth, change and transformation for everyone they met. We found people who could say anything and everything to each other, without fear of reprisal or abandonment. And we found people actively co-creating a new culture that started and ended with the infinite value of each human being.

Despite outward appearances, it was no accident that I found these people, that I chose this life, and that I choose to live it forever. The hungers and ideals that led me here have been present all along. Even when lost in the middle of a wilderness, a compass still turns true. Looking back now, it is easy to see the bends in the road that brought me here, each one taking me a step closer to my heart's desire. It may not be the life for everyone, but it is my life, and it is whole.

Chapter 6

Try Something New!

THEY SAY THAT ONE SURE SIGN OF INSANITY is to continually repeat the same behavior yet expect different results. I heard an odd story on the news that illustrates this point.

A man was driving by himself along a lonely mountain road. He took a wrong turn, left the road, and became stuck. It was starting to get late, and was turning cold outside. The expert advice for this situation, in these parts, was to stay in your car and wait for someone to come along. Better to wait for help than to strike out on your own and expose yourself to the elements.

So the man stayed in his car. During the night it snowed. The next day the man continued to follow the experts' advice, and remained in his vehicle, waiting for help to arrive.

There were only two problems with this strategy: first, the mountain road the man had been on was closed during the winter; second, he had become stuck late in November.

No one came. No one was likely to come. But this did not deter the man. He continued to wait in his vehicle, having nothing to eat except snow. Thirty days after he had pulled from the road, he wrote a letter to his employer, expressing faith that the Lord would deliver him – one way or another. (He didn't seem to care which way it was.) The handwriting was neat, and the words were carefully chosen. As far as anyone could tell from the letter, he still seemed in full possession of all his faculties – still capable of getting out of the car and walking for help, had he chosen to do so.

He remained alive in his car for a total of sixty days, according to medical experts. They didn't find his body until May, when the last of the snow had melted and the road had reopened for the summer. His boss, who was interviewed on the news report, observed that the car still looked like new when it was found. Apparently the man had remained calm through to the very end, with no signs of any agitation – no desperate, clawing attempts to escape.

It has occurred to me, since hearing this report, that many people live their lives in a fashion similar to the way this man ended his. They know they are going to die. The experts tell them to wait quietly, that anything else they could do would be even more dangerous. They make themselves comfortable, isolated, enclosed in familiar surroundings. They wait passively, comforted by their religious belief that whatever happens will be God's will, and that heaven awaits. They bide their time, willing prisoners, feeling so much safer inside their familiar cocoon than they would outside, wandering around in the uncharted wild. Better to stick with what they know, even if it kills them, than face the uncertainty of a risky break for freedom, for life.

This book is for people who have had enough of waiting. It's for humans who are fed up with being told that they have to die. It is for those who are ready to get out of the cocoon –

even if it is cold outside, even if all the experts are telling them to wait patiently, even if they're not sure exactly where they're going.

So if you're one of those content to wait quietly inside the car, then you'll be better off if you just put this book down now, and reach for something more soothing. But if you're tired of eating snow, and ready to strike out in search of something more nourishing, then read on ...

Let's head out together.

Part III

The Decision to Live

This section suggests that life and death are the results of decisions we make, and not things that just happen to us.

Chapter 7. Determine Your Immortality Quotient

Are you immortal? Here's how to find out. Take a straightforward quiz that will determine your IQ (Immortality Quotient).

Chapter 8. Your Desire To Live

Before we discuss whether we can *live forever, we need to determine if we really* want *to. Death has become surprisingly well accepted in civilized society today. I'll expose many forms of social conditioning that prepare us to pack it in after only 70 or 80 years.*

Chapter 9. The Benefits of Your Beliefs

Included here is a discussion of the benefits that a belief in your own physical immortality can have on your life today.

Chapter 10. The Three Major Belief Systems

Our beliefs about death form the deepest foundations of our consciousness. These most fundamental ideas shape the rest of our beliefs about ourselves, and our place in the universe. We'll look at the three basic variations in these belief systems, and analyze the advantages and disadvantages of each.

Chapter 11. Your Test Results Are Back

Another real-life story, this time illustrating the power of our beliefs to make our lives into heavens – or living hells.

Chapter 7

Determine Your Immortality Quotient

How will you know if you become immortal? Perhaps you already are – how could you tell? I've devised a straightforward test that will determine your IQ (Immortality Quotient). Simply answer the following questions as honestly as possible, record your answers, and at the end I'll show you how to tally up your score, and will tell you what it means.

Question Number 1: Are you a helpless victim?

Some people believe that their fate is determined by the stars, by an uncaring deity, or by the circumstances of their birth. These people tend to feel like victims of fate.

Others feel empowered to determine their own destinies. Like the poet William Ernest Henley, they say: "I am the master of my fate; I am the captain of my soul."[17]

Given the self-fulfilling powers of belief, both groups tend to be right. Those who feel like victims tend to wait passively for "fate" to happen to them, and are not happy with the results. Those who feel like they are in charge, on the other hand, take the responsibility to make things happen, and are less likely to complain about the outcome.

Question Number 2: Do you want to die?

Some people avoid an honest answer to this question by saying that they aren't ready to go yet, but are sure they will be prepared when it's "their time."

I can't think of any similar question for which most people would so readily accept such an evasive answer. If my question was, instead, "Do you like chocolate?", what would you think of someone who answered, "I love it now, but I won't be able to stand it in twenty years." This doesn't seem to quite make sense, does it? If you want it now, then how can you be so sure that you will stop wanting it later?

People also confuse themselves with this question by mixing up what they want with what they think they are supposed to do. If you ask an eight-year-old boy at the dinner table if he wants some broccoli, then his honest answer is likely to be "Absolutely not!" If his parents are present, though, and he has been educated on the benefits of eating vegetables, then he may dutifully answer "Yes." Some people feel the same way about death. It may be a bitter pill, but they've been told it is good for them, especially when they reach a certain age. So they say "Yes," when they really mean "No."

Another way of making this question unnecessarily difficult is by assuming that you will someday get so "old" and ill that you will be grateful for death. Or by assuming that all your loved ones will suffer the same fate. This reasoning only makes sense, though, if you accept the limitations of aging. The question is: what do you want? If what you really want is to stay youthful and healthy and alive, then you certainly don't want to die.

Question number 2 is too simple for such complicated answers. If you think you want to die, then you have to ask yourself why you are still here. And if you admit that you don't want to die, then you have to question why you would want to change your answer later.

The Envelope, Please ...

"What," you say, "are those all the questions?"
I told you this was a simple test!
If your answers to both questions were "No," then congratulations – you're immortal! If you're not a helpless victim, and you don't want to die, then you must be immortal: no other answer is logically possible.

Perhaps this was a different kind of test than you were expecting. Maybe you expected to receive some kind of validation as an immortal from an outside agency. If this test reveals you to be immortal, though, then it is not because I, or anyone else, proclaimed you so, but because you've decided so for yourself.

Of course, if you don't like the results, then you can always go back and change either or both of your answers. This, after all, is not the kind of test you only take once. No, this is the kind of examination that you administer to yourself every day, and the only answers that count are the ones you reveal in your everyday actions.

If you're still not sure about your answers, then don't worry. The next two chapters will cover the subjects of these questions in more detail: your desire to live, and the benefits of your beliefs.

Chapter 8

Your Desire To Live

WHEN PEOPLE FIRST HEAR OF PHYSICAL IMMORTALITY, their immediate objections are often practical ones. "That's impossible," they say. "Show me a person who's lived to be 200, and then I'll talk to you."

These pragmatic concerns deserve their just due, but they often seem to mask another issue that is more central. Before we discuss the means, we need to make sure we agree on the ends. Because if you aren't sure you really want to live forever, then it's pointless to discuss techniques for doing so.

Voices From The Past

I am not much of a religious authority, but my attention has been drawn to a number of verses from the Bible. After letting these words sink into me, I have gotten in touch with a feeling from them that has surprised me. This new feeling has nothing to do with anything I learned in Sunday school. Neither does it depend upon any special respect for the Bible as a sacred text (something I have never felt), or upon the acceptance of a Judaic-Christian belief system. What I have found in these Biblical quotations is a special feeling that seems quite absent from modern society: a feeling about life and death. Through these words, echoing across the centuries, I feel an awakening passion that somehow seems to have been lost, even among religions that revere these words as holy yet today.

Let me start with a couple of quotations I've already mentioned in an earlier chapter.

> The last enemy that shall be destroyed is death.[18]
>
> — 1 Corinthians 15:26

Note that death is referred to as an "enemy," and that it is to be "destroyed" – pretty strong language. We civilized humans of the 20TH century often speak disparagingly about individual deaths, but it is hard to find a modern example of this attitude towards death in general.

> Yea, his soul draweth near unto the grave, and his life to the destroyers.
>
> If there be a messenger with him, an interpreter, one among a thousand, to shew unto man his uprightness.
>
> Then he is gracious unto him, and saith: Deliver him from going down to the pit: I have found a ransom.[19]
>
> — Job 33:22–24

Here the powers of death are referred to as "the destroyers," and dying is spoken of as "going down to the pit." Not very pleasant imagery. No mention here of an afterlife, or of the friendly light of modern near-death experiences.

> For he hath looked down from the height of his sanctuary; from heaven did the Lord behold the earth;
>
> To hear the groaning of the prisoner; to loose those that are appointed to death;[20]
>
> — Psalms 102:19–20

Our society today doesn't seem to have much to say about the "groaning of the prisoner," or any desire to "loose those that are appointed to death." Judging from our silence on the subject, it would seem that death has become pretty well accepted as a fact of life.

> I will ransom them from the power of the grave; I will redeem them from death: O death, I will be thy plagues; O grave, I will be thy destruction: repentance shall be hid from mine eyes.[21]
>
> — Hosea 13:14

Notice that this condemnation of death includes no qualifications of any kind: no references to violence, or to any particular kinds of death, or to the ages of those who are dying. There is no distinction made between the accidental death of a child and the quiet passing of a senior citizen. This feeling for the horror of death is absolute, unmitigated. It is death, the phenomenon, that is being condemned, and not a particular set of circumstances.

> Behold, I shew you a mystery; we shall not all sleep, but we shall all be changed,
>
> In a moment, in the twinkling of an eye, at the last trump: for the trumpet shall sound, and the dead shall be raised incorruptible, and we shall be changed.
>
> For this corruptible must put on incorruption, and this mortal must put on immortality.[22]
>
> — 1 Corinthians 15:51–53

The more I read these words, the more one thing becomes increasingly clear: the "how" of immortality was as much a mystery for these people as it often is today, but this did not diminish their desire for an unending life of the flesh. These people felt the awful imposition of death, and hungered for an end to it. They didn't know all the details of how this was going to happen, but this didn't stop them from feeling the hunger.

What has happened to this feeling? Despite the vast media barrage that we are subject to daily, I don't hear many complaints about death. Individual deaths are present everywhere in the media, yet there are few if any objections to death as a general phenomenon.

So, if you have questions about how we can achieve immortality, then I am eager to sit down and talk about them – but first we must answer another, more pressing question: what has ever happened to the desire for it?

The "Right to Die" Movement

There is a growing feeling today that people should have the right to commit suicide, and that other people should have the right to help them. Many are adamant that such assisted suicides are a humane practice, especially for those who are old and hopelessly ill. Others feel equally strongly that such a practice is nothing short of murder, no matter how willing the victim. That this "right to die" movement has caused such controversy is a good indication of the tremendous conflicts present in our society around the subject of death.

This recent movement is really an outgrowth of another one, though: one that is older and more firmly established, and less controversial. This larger movement advocates the belief that it is "right to die" – that death, all in all, is a good thing. Listen, for example, to this statement from one of the most widely respected gerontologists in the US.

> After years of thinking about these kinds of issues, I've decided that there is only one objective that is both practical and desirable and that is to strive for maximum human life expectation by eliminating the present leading causes of death. I see no value to society or to the individual in seeking to slow or stop the aging process or to achieve immortality.[23]
>
> — Leonard Hayflick, Ph.D.

This last sentence, in particular, seems extraordinary. There is "no value" – even "to the individual" – in seeking to slow the aging process. What a clear declaration, from one of our leading researchers in the field of aging, that aging and death are morally right.

If this attitude seems acceptable to you, or you can recognize it as one widely held by others, then this should be seen as a sign of this movement's success. If you think that people have always felt like this, and that no change has taken place, then you should return to the Biblical verses cited above.

Something has happened to us. Somewhere along the line, our society has convinced most of its members that death is no great loss. Somehow, we have become accustomed to death, have accepted it as natural, and have become numb to its horrors. We no longer speak of it as an enemy – it has become an old friend. Most of us have suppressed the desire for immortality, without even being aware that we ever had it.

How have we let this happen to us?

Perhaps it is time to start questioning and speaking out against this unspoken assumption that it is "right" to die.

Religion

It is clear, from the verses given above, that many of the contributors to the Bible were talking about physical immortality – about life in the flesh. As I've already pointed out, though, this is not a subject much discussed in religious circles these days. Modern religions – and not just Christian ones – prefer to talk about spiritual eternity. Death is seen as a gateway to a better world.

Christians talk about heaven. Hindus speak of reincarnation. New age believers describe an ascension to a spiritual plane of existence. All of them see life here on earth as limited, and see death as a release to a better place. Hidden amidst the great diversity of available religions is an unspoken agreement: this life here on earth is just a stepping stone to our ultimate destination.

This well-nigh universal belief in an afterlife has helped to make death seem not only palatable, but actually attractive.

Humanity deserves some fresh options, some core belief systems that depict life on earth as desirable and maintainable.

Government

The past few hundred years have seen the predominant form of human government change from monarchy to democracy. The change, of course, has been for the better in most ways. One of the unfortunate byproducts of this trend, however, has been to insulate us from the effects of human death. The democratic form of government has decreased our reliance on individual human beings, and in so doing has contributed to the idea that people are disposable.

It used to be that a ruler had absolute authority, and reigned until his death. When one leader died, and a new one took his place, then the conditions of the state's citizens could change utterly, for better or for worse. The new king might be terrible – but at least you could say that he made a difference.

Our modern forms of government, however, seem bent on creating institutions that do not depend on people. Constitutions limit the powers of our elected leaders. Media coverage of elections effectively filters out "extremists" who might make any substantive changes. Checks and balances between different branches of government, and different legislative groups, create a gridlock that prevents any meaningful action from being taken. Limits on the length of terms, and the numbers of terms, ensure that office holders will leave on a regular basis, preventing the electorate from becoming too attached to any one individual.

We have succeeded in protecting ourselves from abuse by the worst sort of leaders: those who show flagrant disregard for the good of their subjects. We have done so, though, only by creating governments that run themselves, in which the institutions are more important than the people – in which the people are generally interchangeable cogs in a vast machine.

It's time to start putting the emphasis back on the importance of individual people, and decreasing our reliance on impersonal institutions.

Business

The corporation is the standard form of modern business. Other forms exist, like the sole proprietorship and the partnership, but they are reserved for smaller enterprises. To be big, you must be a corporation.

The corporate form of business, though, is designed expressly to ensure that the business can outlast any of its individual participants. Corporate ownership is divided among a number of shareholders. Shares are designed to be easily transferred from one individual to another. Shareholders elect boards of directors, who in turn appoint Chief Executive Officers. (And the tenure of your average CEO these days would make a term-limited political office look like a relatively secure position.)

Personnel offices have become Human Resource organizations (the old name made it seem too much as if there were real people involved). Members of these organizations write job titles and descriptions that make the inhabitants of the positions described seem interchangeable. These modern businesses go to great lengths to avoid dependence on particular individuals. (And Scott Adams, author of the *Dilbert* comic strip, gets more popular every day by exposing the idiocy lurking just beneath the surface of these gleaming facades.)

I remember being shocked a few years ago when I read an obituary of a great industrial leader. He was a man who had made a great impact on my life, but whom I had never known existed: the founder of the Honda Motor Company. I had owned Honda automobiles for years, but it had never before occurred to me that the founder of the company was still alive. I had assumed, I guess, that if such a person ever existed, he was by now long gone, like Henry Ford and the other industrial giants who had started the once-great American auto companies.

As I let the fact of this man's recent existence sink in on me, I began to wonder. Could it be that the "real" reason why the Japanese auto industry had outpaced its US counterpart had been overlooked? Could the Japanese companies have forged ahead because they were still commandeered by real people? Could they have succeeded because they were still being run by the same individuals who had demonstrated the necessary drive to have built them in the first place?

We have built a society in which institutions outlast people. We have created and fostered the myth that these institutions can grow and thrive in these conditions, unaffected by human dying. Once again, we have found ways to accommodate ourselves to death.

Let's stop kidding ourselves – it's the people that make a business succeed, and not the other way around.

Aging

The first thing to note about old age is that more people are living long enough to experience it than ever before. Our medical systems have focused almost all their energies on corrective procedures, and little if any energy on prevention and general wellness. As a result, they have tended to create growing numbers of "senior citizens" who are not really healthy, but who manage to stay alive. Governments and privately funded insurance plans pour millions of dollars into averting one life-threatening catastrophe after another, yet often spend not one thin dime on anything to actually build wellness.

As a result of all this, we have created a model of aging that makes death seem attractive. By the time someone actually dies, they have been struggling to live for so long – generally with failing health, a dwindling bank balance, and a severely diminished quality of life – that everyone is relieved. Mourning is minimal, since the person who actually would have been missed had been eroded beyond recognition long ago.

Retirement is another great way of accommodating death. Mandatory retirement regulations are gradually being eased, but this is only because they are no longer needed – the carrots are working so well that the sticks are no longer needed. Social security, pension plans, IRAs, Keoghs and other financial tools have made it seem almost foolish to continue working beyond the age of 65, at the very latest. General societal conditioning has also made retirement seem like a welcome reward for so many years of hard work.

Retirement makes death seem easier in several ways. It allows everyone to plan for the retiree's departure from the workplace, so as not to disrupt productivity. It minimizes mourning, since the beginning of retirement is a cause for celebration, not sorrow. Then, when the retiree does finally die, they are already replaced and forgotten.

For the retiree, it is obvious that retirement is the beginning of the end. Their income is now fixed if they are lucky, gradually decreasing otherwise. They have no great passions left to satisfy. They amuse themselves for a few years, then gradually pass into oblivion.

Our society has clearly created a standard life cycle that gradually but inexorably prepares us for death. It goes as follows.

Youth: You are raised by your parents.

College and Single Life (optional): You have a brief taste of relative freedom while you are being prepared for the next phase.

Marriage and Children: You start your own family.

Parenting: You work hard to provide for your growing, and increasingly expensive family. Most of your social interaction is with your family and your coworkers.

Mid-Life Crisis: You start to realize where all this is headed, and try desperately to wriggle off the hook.

The Empty Nest: Your children move out and start their own families, ending their dependence on you. By now, you have generally accomplished everything in your chosen career that you are ever likely to. Without a family to raise, and without any career goals, your work seems increasingly meaningless.

Retirement: You joyously end the tyranny of meaningless work and begin the "golden years."

Old Age: Your family no longer needs you. Your coworkers no longer remember you. The medical system has made enough money from you. Your savings are running out, without any possible source of replenishment. Your health is failing.

Death: What a relief!

Is it any wonder that so few people have any interest in immortality? Our whole lives have been programmed around death! What would we do without it?

Maybe if we start living our lives as if we expected to live forever, we can start putting some more life in our years, as well as add more years to our lives.

Science

Most traditional scientists believe in and promote the absolute inevitability of death, despite the absence of any comprehensive theory to explain it. As a result, most people are convinced that death is an unavoidable decree issued by some basic scientific principle. To question death seems as stupid as questioning gravity, and no one wants to appear stupid.

Before the advent of science, people believed in the possibility of change. They knew how things had been up to that point, but they had no reason to believe that they could not be different. Even if they believed in an omnipotent god, they at least believed in a god who could be beseeched, and who could change his mind.

Science has ended all that. The great unspoken message of modern science is that things are the way they are because of universal, immutable natural laws. Death is presented as being one of these laws (even though we have no scientific evidence that it is). The scientists are the judicial system for these laws. They can interpret them, but they cannot change them. The legislature is not in session, and is not likely to return any time soon. The laws cannot be changed. We may as well learn to live with them.

Science has validated death, and made it seem like we can hope for nothing better.

Let's wake up to the fact that there is more science out there to be found, at the same time realizing that nothing yet discovered places any necessary limits on our longevity.

Environmental Concerns

There is mounting evidence that the human race is rapidly causing vast damage to our fragile planet. In only a few decades, we have all become aware that we are depleting and destroying many of the earth's natural resources. Entire species are being exterminated at a tremendous rate. Our water and air are polluted. The atmosphere's ozone layer is developing holes, exposing humans and other species to more intense solar radiation. The list goes on and on.

The overall impression left by all of this is that there are already too many people alive for the planet to handle. Additional life extension for our species – let alone immortality – seems to be adding insult to injury.

For the first time in the history of the human race, we have become apologetic about being alive.

We need to start taking responsibility for our power, so that we can once again take pride in it.

Mass Media

There are many examples I could give of the mass media's attitudes towards life and death, but I think the most telling is a recent children's film: *The Lion King*.

You may protest that this movie is only mindless entertainment, and does not have any deep message. I do not agree. Every story has a theme. If this story's theme is difficult to detect, it is partly because it is so well accepted by society that it is not noticed.

The movie is about the "great circle of life." This phrase is unfinished, though, because the circle is incomplete without death. It is only death that keeps life going in circles, endlessly repeating itself.

If death is missing from this key phrase, it is certainly not from the story. The movie begins with a lion who is the ruler of a happy animal kingdom. He is killed early on. His son mourns his death. The conflict is resolved, however, when the son reaches maturity, becomes just like his father, takes over the throne and starts his own family. Everything is just as it was, and everyone is happy again. The great circle of live has completed another revolution.

When stripped of its cheerful ornamentation and reduced to its essentials, the message of this movie is chillingly clear. Death looks horrible, but it is really only part of the great circle of life. Parents die, but it is really OK, because they are replaceable and hence dispensable. No one individual has any lasting value. One generation replaces another, and nothing is lost.

If you think that I have singled out one movie that is different from all the rest, then try watching *Bambi* again. Once you become aware of this sort of theme, it becomes disturbingly evident throughout our culture.

Is it any wonder that most of us accept death so willingly, when the programming starts at such a young age? We are taught to accept death before we are even old enough to question it.

We need to acknowledge the infinite value of every human life, and stop acting as if we were no more than beasts of the field.

A Desire to Live

If you ask most people whether they want to live, they will reply, "Why yes, of course – doesn't everybody?"

The sad truth is that not everyone does. Many facets of our culture have conspired to make us feel that it is "right to die." This is why the subject of physical immortality stirs antagonism in some, and leaves others feeling only a mild academic interest.

It is not too late. We can still reclaim our birthright. It is not too late to get excited about living. We can still rediscover the infinite, inexhaustible value of every person alive. It is not too late to feel our aliveness, the wonderful inspiration of living flesh. We can still rekindle the passion that made us who we are.

We can pursue immortality. But questions of how to live forever are idle ones unless we can first agree that we really want to.

Chapter 9

The Benefits of Your Beliefs

WHEN DETERMINING YOUR IMMORTALITY QUOTIENT, I asked you whether you were a helpless victim. I later said that, no matter what your answer, your beliefs would likely prove you right.

But are your beliefs really relevant? The idea that your beliefs can shape your reality is a relatively new one in our modern culture. Is this just an example of fuzzy thinking, more wish-fulfillment than reality, or is there any substance to it?

More and more evidence is showing that our beliefs really can help determine our reality, and even our life expectancy. Investigators at Brown University found that optimism does make a difference. After analyzing data on over 1,300 people aged 70 or more, they found that those who viewed old age as the main source of their health problems were 78% more likely to die, compared to those who did not blame their ills on their age. The researchers concluded that people who blamed their troubles on old age tended not to take as good care of themselves, compared to those who had only themselves to blame.[24]

A survey done by *Prevention* magazine is even more interesting.²⁵ Readers were asked a number of questions about their beliefs. They were also asked numerous questions about their health and sense of well-being.

Over 12,000 of the magazine's readers responded to the survey. Analysis of their answers revealed that people with the following seven beliefs tended to feel healthier, more energetic, and happier than those with different beliefs. Here are the beliefs that made the biggest difference to these *Prevention* readers.

1. Optimism

2. Faith in a Higher Power

3. A Focus on the Future

4. Belief in the Goodness of People

5. A Sense of Trust

6. A Feeling of Control Over One's Life

7. A Feeling of Control Over One's Health

The *Prevention* survey pointed out that it was necessary for the respondents to have at least six out of these seven beliefs, in order to reap the most benefits.

What I can't understand is how a person can hold even one of these beliefs, without also having a belief in the possibility of their own personal immortality.

Let's look at these key attitudes again.

1. How optimistic can you be if you believe yourself headed for certain death and destruction?

2. Faith in a higher power is important because it bestows a belief in the eternal, a belief also bestowed by a belief in physical immortality.

3. How far in the future can you focus, especially as you get older, if you feel that most of your life is behind you?

4. It's difficult to trust in the goodness of people, if you also think that everyone you know will eventually leave you, if not in life than in death.

5. How can you trust in a universe that you think is out to get you?

6. How can you feel in control of your life, if you feel that it could end arbitrarily at any moment?

7. How can you feel in control of your health, if you also feel that you must inevitably grow old and infirm through aging?

More and more research is showing that beliefs really do make a difference in our lives. Even with the constrained belief in a limited number of years, people have shown themselves to be happier and healthier, and to actually live longer, if they hold a certain positive set of beliefs.

How much more could be achieved with a real, unrestrained, unlimited sense of optimism?

The reader is definitely advised to please *do* try this at home.

Chapter 10

The Three Major Belief Systems

OUR BELIEFS ABOUT DEATH are the most fundamental beliefs that we hold. They form the foundation of all else that we consider true. At this most basic level, then, it is good to realize that there are only three possible belief systems.

1. Death is Final and Inevitable

This sort of belief is always characterized by cynicism and despair. These sorts of beliefs are most often expressed by way of bumper stickers and T-shirts. Some examples follow.

He who dies with the most toys wins.

Help! There's some blood in my alcohol stream.
Life is short. Drink hard.

Eat healthy, exercise and *die anyway!*

Many authors have pointed out the difficulties of living a full and meaningful life if we also harbor a belief in our own mortality. Dr. Paul Pearsall, psychiatrist and best-selling author of *Super Marital Sex* and *Superimmunity,* made these comments.

> If death means nothing but an end, how could there be any joy in living? ... we fool ourselves if we think that the stoic acceptance of our passing will ever be acceptable to the human psyche.[26]
>
> — Paul Pearsall, Ph.D.

Any belief in the finality of death will ultimately make us feel cynical and hopeless.

2. Death is a Transition to an Afterlife

This second approach to death is the one characteristic of religion. All modern religions seem to offer a consoling belief in some sort of afterlife.

In the *Prevention* survey cited earlier, the magazine showed that one of the beliefs highly correlated with exceptional health was a strong belief in a higher power. In explaining this connection, the article offered the following comment.

> Faith in an eternal or life-transcending force is a supremely soothing belief. It disconnects unhealthy logic and worries.[27]
>
> — Herbert Benson, MD

Others have also observed the connection between human well being and a belief in some sort of life after death.

> Our mental health may depend on the acceptance of death, but super joy and extraordinary mental hardiness depend on seeing death as a natural transition to another state of existence.[28]
>
> — Paul Pearsall, Ph.D.

Unfortunately, religious beliefs also bring other baggage with them. Any sort of belief in a spiritual afterlife inevitably brings some sort of separation between physical and spiritual existence. The worst forms of such beliefs motivate terrorists who think that suicide bombings will bring them closer to God. Other religious beliefs promote a sense of detachment from the physical world, and a devaluing of physical life in favor of the spiritual.

Some of these spiritual beliefs are healthier than others. Some may even be quite supportive of human existence. Once we open the door to religion, though, we lose control of what form it takes. Since there is no more rational basis for one religious belief than another, there is no way for humanity to converge on a single religious belief system. Belief in an afterlife inevitably leads us to the modern tower of Babel that we face today, with different cultures holding radically different beliefs, and with no way to reconcile them.

Humanity has taken spiritual beliefs to the end of the line. They will not take us any farther. There is no way to follow the path of religion, without creating the discord we see today, and without creating some sort of split between the physical and the spiritual.

3. Physical Immortality

A belief in human physical immortality is the only way out of this dilemma. It is the only other alternative to the finality of death, and to the confusion of religion.

A belief in the possibility of living forever allows us to create lives full of hope, excitement, passion and wholeness.

It's Up To Us

All of humanity's intricate belief systems can be placed into one of these three categories. And, no matter what other beliefs are laid on top of these foundations, they remain fundamentally the same, with the same appeals and pitfalls.

Which belief we choose is up to us. But once we make this fundamental decision, we have to accept the additional freight that comes with each one.

Which of these three belief systems have you chosen, and what consequences ensue from this most fundamental decision?

Chapter 11

Your Test Results Are Back

I ONCE READ A NEWSPAPER ARTICLE that made some telling points about the consequences of the belief systems we choose. To me, at least, it speaks volumes about the massive contradictions our society contains when it approaches the subjects of life and death.

Let me start by saying I've noticed two common reactions to news of the possibility of physical immortality. One is disbelief: a doomed resignation to the death sentence seemingly imposed upon us. Another is bewilderment: a confusion about what the prospect of eventual immortality might have to do with the way we live our lives today. I think that the story I'm about to tell shows the lie in both reactions.

The tale begins with a woman worrying that she might have been infected with AIDS. She had received a blood transfusion ten years earlier, and is now concerned that the deadly virus might have been transmitted to her. The woman decides to relieve her anxiety by having herself tested. But when her results come back, the diagnosis confirms her worst fears: she is HIV-positive.

Her life now takes a turn for the worst. Afraid of passing the infection on, she no longer allows her three children to hug her. Her dirty dishes are washed with bleach after every meal, to prevent passing the contagion to the rest of her family. She begins taking a medication that leaves her feeling nauseous and weak. Sure that she has little time left, she transfers legal custody for her children to her mother. Finally, after two years of this living hell, she returns to her home town, prepared to take her own life when the illness becomes too much for her to bear.

So far, you might be thinking, this story is fairly unremarkable, similar in general outline, if not in detail, to thousands of others. But wait – a remarkable twist follows, one worthy of a short story by O. Henry. Perhaps growing suspicious after displaying a remarkable lack of symptoms (the account I read is vague on this point), the woman decides to have herself tested again. This test comes back negative. It turns out that her original test results had been misdiagnosed. She is not now, nor was she ever, HIV-positive. Outraged over her needless suffering, she sues everyone involved with the original test, and is eventually awarded over half a million dollars by a jury.

So what does this story have to do with physical immortality? Let me reduce the story to its bare bones. Supposedly knowledgeable authorities tell a person that she is dying. Believing them without question, her life is subsequently ruined – not by the disease she supposedly has, but by her unquestioning belief that she is doomed. Finally, it becomes clear to everyone that the authorities were simply and collectively wrong. The pain and suffering she has endured are so real that a jury of her peers awards her a huge sum of money in compensation.

What I find most remarkable about this story is that, when reduced to its simplest elements, it could be told by almost everyone. The authorities inform all of us that we are suffering from a terminal illness: life. As a result, people distance themselves from their loved ones, anticipating the eventual separation of death. People make preparations for their supposedly inevitable demise. As a result, their lives are dominated more by death than by life.

And yet, even though most people will believe the story I have told without question, they will still refuse to believe that the same story might apply to them. They will have a hard time accepting that our common human diagnosis might be in error, and will find it difficult to understand what a belief in their own eventual demise could have to do with their life today.

This book is your personal wake-up call. Your new test results are back. I'm here to tell you that you have been misdiagnosed. Forget what the experts told you. I have a new prognosis for you: unlimited life.

Welcome to the land of the living.

Part IV

How To Live Forever

Chapter 12. The Fifteen Minimum Requirements

What would it take for a human being to live forever? This part of the book reveals what I call the fifteen minimum requirements for physical immortality. I believe that these techniques are bound to improve your life today, and offer real hope of extending our lives indefinitely.

Chapter 12

The Fifteen Minimum Requirements

WHAT DO YOU HAVE TO DO IN ORDER TO LIVE FOREVER? Many people have strong preconceptions about the sort of answer they expect to this question. They think it will come in the form of a "silver bullet" – some single, magical secret, like Ponce de León's Fountain of Youth. Many expect it to be some long-forgotten technique – the "secrets of the ancients." Others look forward to particular techniques, or some special substance to ingest.

I see things a little differently. First, I don't have any single answer. Second, I don't claim to have all the answers. Third, I am talking about doing something new, and believe that "ancient secrets" are not enough. Fourth, I have no rigid set of techniques or dietary recommendations to recommend.

In other words, I do not have any easy recipe that is guaranteed to bring you physical immortality.

What I have to offer, instead, amounts to a set of minimum requirements. Instead of starting with the widespread assumption that people die because they are supposed to, I have taken the opposite view – that there are specific causes for death. What I have identified, then, are a number of practices, traits and attitudes that seem to lead to death. When reversed, their opposites seem to promote life.

As you will see, these minimum requirements are general precepts. No one can precisely measure to what degree you are living in accordance with these principles. It is up to you to incorporate these guidelines into your life as best you can.

I want to stress, however, that these are *all* part of the minimum requirements for living forever. This is not a case where you can pick the requirement that seems easiest and ignore the rest. This is not a test on which a score of 70% will earn you a passing grade. Nor is this a menu that permits substitutions, allowing you to choose the baked potato over the rice pilaf. To the best of my knowledge, physical immortality requires us to meet each and every one of these requirements, as a minimum.

1. Go With Your Aliveness

Daily living offers us an almost continuous series of choices between life and death, between living and dying. It is important that we make these choices consciously, and that we consistently choose life and living.

Are you making payments on a life insurance policy? Do you have a last will and testament? Have you purchased a burial plot? Realize that these are all choices made by you, and that these choices have consequences. You cannot choose death in one area of your life, and then pretend to choose life in another. Your body is smart enough to know the difference.

2. Put People First

It is customary, especially in modern Western societies, to place a high value on human life. It may come as a bit of a shock, then, to realize that although people often place high on our list of priorities, they rarely if ever come first.

Actually, human values fall into a fairly predictable order, once we realize the strong correlation between the longevity of an item and its perceived worth. Abstractions, such as truth, justice, and moral codes, generally come first, since they can theoretically last forever. Long-lived human products – works of art, nations, modern corporations and the like – tend to be next, since they may not last forever, but can easily outlast any single human individual. People come next, followed by everything else destined to last a lesser number of years.

If we are serious about physical immortality, then we will have to change this customary order of things. If people are to live forever, then we must make individual human beings – not humanity as a whole, nor some special group of "gifted" people – the most important thing in the universe.

It may take some practice to make your next door neighbor more important than an abstract principle – democracy, for example – but it is essential. As long as any member of our species is disposable, then physical immortality can have no possible justification, in your own mind or in anyone else's. If limits can be placed on the value of any living human being, then none of us are safe. For sooner or later, under certain conditions, all of us will reach the same limits, and will be judged to be disposable. It is only when we view our human worth as something intrinsic to our aliveness, that we will genuinely be able to see all people as deserving to live forever.

3. Get Physical

Humankind has been heavily conditioned to think of eternity in spiritual terms. This is why it is often necessary to qualify the term "immortality" with the word "physical." Even then, people often assume that the subject is some form of mental or spiritual mastery of the body.

There is much good advice available today on the care and maintenance of the human body. There is information on supplements, nutrition, diet and exercise, to name a few of the basics. Although I don't endorse any specific program or practice, I do strongly recommend that people take good care of themselves physically. It is clear, for example, that smoking is bad for your health, and is not consistent with physical immortality. Obesity is also harmful. Diets high in saturated fats are not conducive to healthful living.

I've named only a few obvious examples. What's important, though, is not for you to get in touch with what I think. Instead, you need to get in touch with your own body, to take responsibility for your own health, and to do all you can to make yourself physically healthy. This need not be hard or oppressive. It is fun and exciting to have a healthy body!

4. Get Real

Some people mistakenly identify physical immortality with wishful thinking. They think that if we look at the world through rose-colored glasses, all the weeds in our garden will magically turn into beautiful flowers.

I am not telling anyone to ignore reality. On the contrary, I encourage people to get in better touch with it! If you are experiencing a medical problem, or a challenge in your health, then I am *not* telling you to stick your head in the sand and hope it will go away. Instead, I encourage you to seek the best medical care available, and to take action quickly.

Reality does not just come in the form of serious problems, though. Reality is available continuously, in the form of our feelings, our experiences and our actions. Get in touch with it. Reality is offering all of us continuous feedback about the success of our living. Pay it constant heed. If your life is not all that you want for yourself, then do something different.

5. Take 100% Responsibility

Are you totally responsible for all facets of your life? If not, then who is? And if you're not responsible for it, then how can you hope to change it?

Taking responsibility for your life is the difference between taking positive, constructive action and taking the day off. If you hold yourself responsible, then you will work to improve your situation. If you consider someone else responsible, then you will sink to whining and complaining about your plight, or passively accepting it.

Nothing in this world has been deemed so inevitable as death. So, if you leave open any possibility that there is a part of your life for which you are not responsible, then death will certainly creep into that opening.

Close the door. Take responsibility for all of it. Make the decision to live, and let nothing stop you from living fully.

6. Identify Root Causes

Many people, especially as they get older, tend to dismiss physical problems as being caused by aging. Once a patient hits 40, doctors begin responding to their ailments by saying, "Oh, well, that's just part of getting old." People adjust their expectations downward, and stop looking for the real causes of their problems.

If we are to live forever, then we must get to the roots of problems when they come up. We can't take any negative situations in our lives for granted. We must be willing to explore all our options, make decisions about what we want for ourselves, and take positive actions to get back on the right track.

7. Close All The Exits To Death

Humanity's many and varied religions have all agreed on one thing – they all offer hope of some form of life after death. Even in the United States, a country that has prided itself on offering freedom of religion, it has been difficult to find freedom *from* religion. This is perhaps why, even though the separation of church and state is a basic principle on which the US government is founded, its currency still bears the inscription, "In God We Trust." The implication seems to be that you are free to believe in any sort of God you choose – so long as you believe in some sort.

All of these religions have made it easy to believe – consciously or otherwise – that there is some better place awaiting us after death. Unfortunately, the same beliefs have also made it difficult to commit ourselves fully here, in this life, on this earth, and in this body. We have felt like – and acted like – tenants living in a home that belongs to someone else. We have maintained it well enough to make ourselves comfortable, perhaps, but have avoided making any long-term investments in the place.

As long as you harbor any hope that there is some better place to live, then you will need an emergency exit from this life that you can take when things get too tough. As long as you consider your current residence to be only a stop along the way, then you will leave open a back door from your earthly existence. Do whatever it takes to close the door, to lock it, and to nail it shut! Fully commit yourself to staying here – don't leave yourself any outs.

8. Make Growth A Way Of Life

Living forever does not make any sense if we are talking about eternal stagnation. Life, at its core, is all about growth. The point at which we cease to grow is also the point at which we begin to die. Besides, if we have to stop growing, then who would want to live forever?

Unfortunately, the modern model for human life calls for most growth to end by the time a person reaches what is commonly called "middle age." By then, you are supposed to be a fully realized human being, and are expected to stay that way until you die. Is it any surprise, then, that physical decline usually begins around the same time?

Death is not inevitable, but evolution is. Death has been a mechanism, an important cog in the machinery of Darwinian evolution. And even though social change now happens much faster than genetic change, the replacing of one generation by another has itself come to play an important role in the machinery of our cultural evolution. We don't expect our elders to change their ways, but continually look to our youth to pioneer new trends in fashion, in the arts, in science and in government.

If we are to stop dying, then we must begin to evolve on our two feet. We must change and grow as we live, never ending, never reaching or even trying for a state of perfection, but always growing into something new.

9. Accept Your Whole Self

Humanity has traditionally split its identity into shattered splinters of its whole self. We have created a division between our spiritual selves and our physical selves, between mind and body, between emotion and reason, between male and female, God and Devil.

The truth is that each one of us is an organic whole that is bigger, and more integrated, than any of these fragmented perceptions. Your spiritual self is not separate from your physical body – it is a manifestation of it. Your mind is not a grayish organ that is confined to your cranium – your body is mind all over. Your emotions are not some aberrant impulses that need to be controlled by your reason – your feelings and your thoughts are inseparable. Your sensual feelings, your personality, and your attitudes are not rigidly governed by your sexual equipment – you are a whole that includes male and female, no matter how you are equipped. And there is no part of you that is more divine than any other.

We need all of ourselves to live forever. So long as you deny or suppress any part of your aliveness, then you are forcing yourself to function as a cripple, without the benefit of all your limbs and organs. So long as you continue to see any part of yourself as inferior, any component as worthy of anything less than eternity, then you are casting a death sentence on your entire organism.

10. Become a Vital Part of a Greater Whole

No matter how great and wonderful you become, there are limits to your own personal growth and expansion. You can be everything that you are – but you will never be who I am.

The wonderful truth is that we need each other – often more than we like to admit. We need each other's different perspectives, we need the stimulation of each other, we need the warm physical contact of other people. As individual human beings, any one of us is limited and small in many ways. But as part of a greater whole – part of humanity, part of life on earth, and part of the universe – we have no limits at all.

This does not mean, though, that our own individuality is to become lost in a greater whole. It is not size that makes the whole greater – it is the combination of the many unique contributions made by each individual. Each person is as unique and irreplaceable as they allow themselves to be.

11. Express Your Heart's Desire

It is one thing to silently believe everything that I am saying. It is another to express it to another human being, to give voice to it, to sing it, to scream it if necessary. Do not take lightly the human gift of language, or the voice with which to express it. Our words do make a difference. We need to speak our dreams and visions into reality – and not by speaking into a void, but by speaking them to another person, or to a group of people. We need to make our words flesh.

12. Choose Your Genetics Carefully

We are taught to be proud of our genetic heritage. We are trained to believe in the importance of family, to remember that "blood is thicker than water." Our societies stress the importance of carrying on the family name. We look eagerly at our newborn children, and rejoice at each freshly discovered genetic trait they share with us – the characteristic hair, the aristocratic nose, or the endearing shape of the mouth. Some of us have even been taught to be proud of our inherited genetic weaknesses, reflective as they are of our ancestral lines.

Our families and our genetics can certainly be beneficial to us. If we are to be physically immortal, though, then it will only be by going beyond the evolutionary mechanism of genetic inheritance. Before you take too much pride in your family tree, remember that blind chance and mutation play a major role in genetic selection, according to Darwin's rules.

By all means, take what is good from your family and your genetics, and cherish the members of your family as precious human beings. But be careful not to take on all the limitations, the prejudices, and the rigidity that are so often created as part of the family structure.

13. Stop Separation

Death and separation seem to go hand-in-hand. Death causes separation, not only in its final violent act, but in the daily detachment from each other caused by the apprehension of death. Our fear of eventual abandonment causes us to pull back from one another, to not fully invest ourselves in one another, to fail to go all the way with each other. We are all looking for people who will never leave us, but are cheated by the specter of death. What good is unconditional love, when we lack unconditional life?

What is perhaps less obvious is that separation also causes death. Separation from those close to us, whether from fear of death or other reasons, deprives us of our very reason for living. Separation between males and females causes oppression and dominance/submission games. Separation between the generations causes alienation and rebellion. Separation based on the color of our skin, our place of birth, or our cultural heritage, causes discrimination, crime and war.

The greatest nutrient that people have been missing in their lives is the nourishment of each other – the touch of flesh, the intimate word, the excitement of our interaction. Separation stifles this flow.

14. Practice Active Creation

Our modern technological societies teach us to be passive consumers. Creation is a professional act reserved for a privileged few, located in some special place like Hollywood. The greatest blessing – and the greatest curse – of modern forms of communication is that they allow millions and even billions of people to become the passive recipients of a single act of creation.

Too many people now think that freedom is a matter of having more cable channels to choose from, more compact discs in their home entertainment center, and more movie theaters in their local mall. The bland sameness of all these diversions, and the vast richness of human experience that goes unrepresented in these various entertainments, seem to go almost unnoticed.

If we are to live forever then we must create something new, something that has never existed before on this planet. And yet creativity is like a muscle that grows stronger the more it is used, more atrophied the less it is exercised. Creation is not something we observe on TV – it is something we must constantly practice in our daily lives, at every level.

There is no such thing as steady-state immortality. Life is a series of acts of creation.

15. Find Some Great Reasons For Living

Many people, when confronted with the possibility of physical immortality, respond not with the question of how, but the question of why. "Why bother? Who would want to live forever, anyway? I'm bored with my life already."

If we are to live forever, then we must have some really great reasons for living. We need some reasons that won't wear out, that won't get old and stale, but that will continue to expand and grow, for all of eternity. And the more of these reasons we have, the better.

I'm fortunate to have a number of great reasons. I don't have room to list them all, but let me name a few. Pauline and Stephen Bowie, who live with me. Charles Paul Brown, Bernadeane Brown, and James Russell Strole. Shmulik and Raya BenDror, in Israel. Clem and Pat Collard, in New Zealand. Egbert Sukop, from Germany. Veronica Pinerua and Andres Bonomie, in Venezuela.

I could go on and on, but the names of the people who are important to me may not mean much to you. What's important to you is the people you have in your life, the people you know you can count on, the ones who will never leave you, the people who make life worth living.

I don't know about you, but I can never have too many of these people in my life. That's one reason why I am writing this – to reach someone like you. We could just be each other's best reasons to live.

Scientific Validation

I cannot offer any scientific proof that adherence to these 15 principles will cause you to live forever. I have said, though, that physical immortality offers humanity a new wholeness. Part of this wholeness is reflected in the way that the means to immortality are also the ends.

If you look back over these 15 principles, you will see that all of them are worthy practices for their own sake. All of them have the power to transform your life today. So even if you don't know for sure that they will enable you to live forever, you should find them worth doing for the difference they will make in your life today.

I believe that there is a strong correlation between quality of life and length of life. By quality of life, I do not necessarily mean a degree of ease or comfort, but a degree of vitality and excitement. If you look over what I call the minimum requirements for immortality, you will see that all of these guidelines will increase your quality of life. And this is something that you should be able to validate for yourself, without having to take my word for it.

I'll cover many of these principles in more detail later in the book.

Part V

Feelings

What does it feel like to be immortal? And what kinds of feelings nourish our immortality? This section talks about the importance of recognizing and nurturing our feelings of being here forever. In this section I talk about what it feels like to look forward to eternity.

Chapter 13. A Forever Kind of Feeling

A feeling of eternity is an essential part of living forever. This is not a complicated feeling. In fact, it is so simple that it is often overlooked.

Chapter 14. Embracing the Unknown

There can never be any guarantees about living forever. So making the commitment to eternity requires us to live beyond our expectations. To live forever, we must be willing to continually explore the unknown.

Chapter 13

A Forever Kind of Feeling

> Death is a very dull, dreary affair, and my advice to you is to have nothing whatever to do with it.
>
> — W. Somerset Maugham

THERE IS A FEELING OF ETERNITY that we are all born (or at least conceived) with. There is nothing complicated about this feeling. It is "just" a feeling of aliveness. It is a feeling of going on. It is a feeling of timelessness. This feeling has no external frame of reference. It is not learned. It comes from within.

As we grow older, we become conscious of the flow of time. We become aware of things that have happened in the past. We anticipate things we expect to happen in the future. We measure our progress by events that approach, reach us, and then pass behind, like street lamps on a dark road. We begin by measuring our progress against the event of our birth. And, at some point, we begin to measure our remaining time against the anticipated event of our death.

Both of these sensations are available to us: this feeling of timelessness, and the awareness of time. It is like riding in a car. If you focus your attention on the car itself, its passengers, and its contents, then you have no sense of movement. If you look out the window, at the scenery whizzing by, then you are conscious of your speed.

Even though both these perspectives are available, they are mutually exclusive. This belief in our mortality, our winding down, our decay, robs us of life. It sends a cold chill up our spine. It numbs and deadens us. This anticipation of our own demise causes us to feel hopeless and paralyzed, like a mouse cornered by a cat.

When we get in touch with our aliveness, though, we lose this sense of time. When we allow ourselves to feel what is going on inside of us, it is a feeling of living. It is a feeling of excitement. This sense of being fully alive warms us all over. It quickens us.

As we experience life, we have to continuously choose. Do we focus our attention on our feeling of aliveness, or on an awareness of aging and growing older?

The Myth of Aging

Many people would tell you that the awareness of aging and growing older is more "real," because it can be measured by objective means. You're bigger now than you were at the age of 10. You may be conscious of other physical changes. Perhaps there is some gray in your hair. Perhaps you are aware of other signs of "aging."

The common view of aging is that it goes on continuously, uncontrollably, and at a uniform rate. Another common view is that getting older inevitably causes physical deterioration.

These are not scientific truths, though. They are myths.

First, we need to realize that we have no precise definition of what we mean by aging. To "age" means "to become old," and "old" means "advanced in years," so one definition of immortality could be to age without end. In this sense, aging is not at all a bad thing.

Another sense of aging, of course, is a collection of negative physical conditions that we associate with getting old. What's important to realize here is that science has no single, comprehensive explanation for these conditions. The popular notion is that there is some simple internal mechanism that accounts for all of these complex external occurrences: graying hair, weakening bones, lower resistance to disease, etc. In truth, science has discovered no such simple mechanism that can account for all of these conditions. Scientifically speaking, there is no single phenomenon that can be called "aging."

Even if we were to concede that there is some process of gradual and general deterioration called aging, science has no convenient way to measure the rate of this progress. Doctors can assess the changes in a number of physical characteristics that take place over relatively long time periods, but this gives us no immediate feedback on how we are doing today. There is no medical device in the world, no scientific instrument, that can tell you the rate at which you are "aging" at this moment. So perhaps you age faster at some times than others. There are stories of people whose hair turned gray overnight – after having been exposed to some terrible shock, or after the start of a war.

On the other hand, you may age more slowly at other times. At some moments, perhaps "aging" stops altogether. At other times, rejuvenation may be working faster than deterioration, so you may actually be "youthing"! We have all seen people who suddenly looked younger, when some great stress was removed from them.

So if we are talking about what is happening to you at any

given moment, there is no objective scientific authority who can state with certainty that you are "aging." So there is no justification for saying that this awareness of aging is "real."

The Reality of Agelessness

What, then, about this feeling of timelessness? If this is some artificially induced mental state, then it is not real either. But what happens if you let go of your knowledge that you are getting older every minute? What if you let yourself really feel what it is like to be alive? You may just discover this feeling of eternity somewhere inside of you! I'm not talking about a feeling that comes from any kind of truth you have been taught. I'm speaking of a feeling that runs beneath the surface of your everyday consciousness, like a hidden stream of water beneath the ground. You can walk right over it every day and never know that it is there. But stop, and dig down a bit, and it springs forth, clear and sweet.

So is this feeling of timelessness real? Most of us have been taught that we cannot trust our feelings, that they are only subjective. But only you can determine the depth of your feelings of agelessness. I can tell you that my own feelings of aliveness, of eternity, of timelessness, are more real than my knowledge of aging. Yet I can choose to focus on either one. I can dwell on signs of aging, and expectations of getting older, or I can focus on this feeling of going on, of being endless, of being unlimited.

Some people say that they get in touch with a feeling of timelessness by focusing on their connection to the cosmos, or to God, or to the infinite intelligence of the universe. All of these techniques may be valuable. And it is true that we are all part of something bigger, that includes other things that do not appear to age as quickly as humans. But it is good to remember that this sense of connection comes from us. These thoughts of eternity come from within. These images of a timeless cosmos are reflections of our own sense of agelessness. We can imagine that this ageless quality is somewhere outside ourselves, but it is more accurate – and more empowering – to acknowledge it as our own.

This feeling of an endless aliveness is so simple that it is easy to overlook, easy to forget. There is not a whole lot to say about it. Yet this feeling of timelessness is the core of physical immortality. Starting from here, we can speak volumes about immortality. But if we ever wander too far from this point, if we ever lose this feeling, then the rest of our words become hollow and empty.

Aging or agelessness. Your choice. See which feels better. And always remember that you have a choice.

Chapter 14

Embracing the Unknown

THERE IS A SUBTLE IMPLICATION OF PHYSICAL IMMORTALITY that is often overlooked. Common interpretations of this state frequently picture immortality as irreversible. Popular stories depict immortals as continuing to live, even with holes blown through them. Immortality is seen as the mirror image of mortality, with eternal life now just as certain as death once was.

The truth, however, is that there are no guarantees. There is no magic elixir that will make you indestructible. There is no power outside of yourself who can say with certainty that you will live forever. So, if you decide to do so anyway, then you have to learn to live with a degree of uncertainty that is foreign to most people. This is the subtle distinction between the two states that is generally missed.

You see, for most people, death is perfectly certain. Because the one thing I can guarantee is: if you believe you will die, you will. So if you are attracted by the idea of a sure thing, then death is pretty hard to resist. It is utterly reliable. It has a perfect track record. You can bank on it.

And most people do. They plan their lives around it. They forecast their longevity and schedule their finances around it. They take out life insurance in case death comes too soon. They put away savings in case it comes a bit later. If it didn't come at all they would have no idea what to do with themselves.

So, as strange as this may sound, many people are very comfortable with the certainty of their own demise. They can count on it, they can plan their lives around it, and all this certainty makes them feel very secure.

Physical immortality, on the other hand, is an entirely different proposition. It is not a sure thing. Neither is it a known state. A life planned around death can resolve itself into a number of well-defined, predictable conditions – being a child, going to school, working for a living, marrying, raising a family of your own, and then retiring. But no one can tell you what it is going to be like to be 200 years old, let alone 2,000. No one. Not me. Not even you. As hard as you may try, you cannot plan an immortal life. All you can do is live it.

So an intrinsic part of embracing physical immortality is embracing the unknown. I use this word "embracing" intentionally. We cannot achieve immortality by putting up with the unknown. We must love this feeling of unknowing. Because living with the unknowable is not just a side effect of living forever, it essentially is living forever. This is what we're talking about. This is the immortal life.

This unknown is not something waiting for us at some far distant point in the future, though. If we are going to get off the freeway to death, then we have to take the next exit. We have to abandon the eight-lane super highway and get lost on the side roads of life today.

The Unknown Universe

A friend of mine recalls a scientific theory he heard as a child. One morning his father was all excited about an article in the science section of the *New York Times*. This piece reported a new theory that our universe was shaped like a bathtub. My friend remembers thinking that this was absolutely stupid, because if the universe was shaped like a bathtub, then what was shaped like the bath*room?*

To say that the universe stops somewhere doesn't make any sense. What would the end of the universe look like? Would there be a sign? Would there be a wall, separating the universe from the nothingness, or the something elseness, beyond?

Let's face it, the universe goes on *forever.* Or, if not the universe, then something does. Something goes on forever, whatever we decide to call it.

This urge to draw a nice, neat border around something and call it complete is a recurring trait in the human race. How else explain the *Biosphere 2* project undertaken in Arizona? Several intrepid adventurers agreed to be locked inside a sealed dome for two years, almost completely isolated from the outside world. Independent scientists saw little in the way of true science to be gained from this project. The sole motivation seemed to be a pure desire to draw a border around a chunk of space and call it complete: a "biosphere." The "2," by the way, was in honor of the earth, supposedly the original model.

Ah, the appeal of a closed system, in which all the components are known, and in endless, perfect balance. Unfortunately, no such system exists. The inhabitants of *Biosphere 2* depended on recurring input from the outside support system (and still they seemed to get continually thinner). The earth depends on the rays of the sun. Every womb has its umbilical cord. All closed systems eventually die, or are birthed, which is another way of saying that every apparently closed system is really part of a larger open system. There is only one true system, and it is an open one, and it is called the universe.

The universe will always be too big for us to get our arms around. The unknown will be always with us. Why fight it?

But the unknown is not patiently waiting for us at the edge of the universe, just as immortality is not reserved for some far distant future. It is here, now.

We are either forever right now, unlimited, free, or we are still marking the way toward our own nothingness. Death is yet another border, another nice neat line saying "here is the end of a universe." Our entire life arranges itself around this known, because this is for sure, this is certain, and we are more comfortable with certainty than aliveness. There are only the two choices. Either we feel the unknown, in every moment of our lives, or we accept this precise line marking the end of our existence.

This Indeterminate Life

Life is inherently unpredictable. If we subscribe to the theory of evolution – and modern science increasingly leaves us little choice in the matter – then we must accept that life did not progress according to some grand plan. All the incredible, amazing varieties of life that exist today happened without any forethought. Even if some infinitely intelligent bystanders had been around at the very beginning, they could not have predicted what course life would take.

What does it mean to embrace the unknown? Not just in 100 years, but now and every day?

First and foremost, it means living from our feelings, and not from our head. Our minds are very good at arranging our lives for us. We can neatly categorize ourselves and others. We can make our lives entirely regular and predictable. We can tell ourselves what it is safe to feel and when, what it is safe to do and with whom. We can use the entertainment media to stimulate our emotions while we are comfortably seated in our home entertainment center. We can rely on the authorities to tell us how to live. Death fits neatly into such a life.

The alternative is to let ourselves fully feel what it is to be alive. This is a life without borders, without restrictions, without limits. This is a life in which we can change jobs and careers when we feel like it. This is a life in which we can move to the other side of the globe. This is a life that goes on even after the children have grown up and moved out. This is a life that includes people who don't fit into the nice, neat categories of friends, family and coworkers. Death has no place in such a life.

To many, this sort of life sounds dangerous and chaotic. And it can be, if it is lived in an image of rebellion against the established norm. This life can also be chaotic if it is lived in a state of disconnection from people who have formerly represented safety and security.

What I am talking about, though, is not a life of chaos. Even when life is unknown and unpredictable, it need not be destructive. We can trust our feelings, when they are connected to the rest of us, and to those around us. We cannot predict them, but we can trust them. And this is what it means to be fully alive: to let ourselves feel everything.

I do not mean that we have to act on every feeling. I do not mean that we have to do everything, to act on every impulse that crosses our minds. But neither, on the other hand, can we rule out certain categories of actions in advance. Because feelings are inextricably tied to actions. If we draw an absolute line around our possible actions, then our feelings will wither away as well. We will become circus elephants, our legs in chains that were once attached to stakes. Now the mere weight of the chain is enough to secure us, since we long ago stopped feeling the desire to test it.

Where will this life of the unknown take us? We do not know – and that is what living forever is all about.

Part VI

Science

The next section looks at the possibility of human physical immortality from a scientific perspective. I point out that the physical and biological sciences have found no fundamental principles that would make immortality impossible. I also explain why I think that the phenomenon of evolution has brought humankind to the brink of a new phase of history, in which immortality is our next logical step.

Chapter 15. Foundations

This chapter establishes a context for our discussion of science and immortality.

Chapter 16. Physics

We take a look at some of the laws of physics, and what they have to say about the possibility of immortality.

Chapter 17. Biology

The life sciences also provide a framework for our ability to extend our lives indefinitely.

Chapter 18. Our Human Nature

What does it mean, not just to be alive, but to be human? And what does being human have to do with the possibility of living forever?

Chapter 19. A Turning Point

The conclusions of this section are twofold: that humanity is at a crossroads in its development, and that physical immortality is an integral part of our better path.

Chapter 15

Foundations

I F WE ARE TO CONSIDER SOMETHING SO EARTH-SHAKING as the possibility of human physical immortality, then we need to start with a good look at the deepest foundations of our belief systems. People have such widely differing beliefs at these most fundamental levels, though, that you may find it distressing for me to raise such issues. Scientists, philosophers and religious leaders have argued about these most basic beliefs throughout all recorded history, and there often seems to be less consensus now than at any point in the past. Like planetary bodies in an expanding universe, the various theories seem to be of an endless number, and moving further apart all the time. Entire volumes have been written expressing particular viewpoints on these most basic questions, and they have often served only to further muddy the waters. So you may well wonder what I can hope to accomplish in this slim volume.

I think we can get quite far, actually, if we start with sensible attitudes towards science and religion.

Science

When I talk about science, I need to make clear that I am talking about fundamental scientific principles. These are the basic beliefs that most "pure" scientists can agree on.

One of the impressive things about science is that scientific beliefs ultimately tend to converge. That is, the experts may argue and disagree for a while, but sooner or later they seem to do enough experiments and gather enough evidence to reach consensus one way or the other. So we can be relatively sure that a large and growing core of scientific belief is actually pretty close to the truth. At the same time, of course, there are various theories that scientists have had ample opportunity to test and find wanting. We can be pretty sure that these theories are indeed false views of reality.

We need to recognize, though, that science is always kind of fuzzy around the edges. New areas of inquiry take a while to become resolved, and scientists may be temporarily quite confused in these areas.

At the farthest extreme, there may be vast areas that are simply outside of established science. Scientists generally don't like to admit this, but just because a theory has not been proven does not mean that it is false. If it has not been extensively tested, or even worse is untestable, then we are free to believe what we like in these unexplored areas. Our rules here should be that our theories are consistent with well-established science, and that the simplest theory that explains a particular phenomenon is generally the best one.

Religion

If we look at religion as a whole, the first thing we notice is something very different from science. Religious beliefs do not seem to converge. If anything, they do the opposite: multiply and diverge. New religions seem to grow like weeds, and well-established religions seem to endlessly subdivide into various denominations and sects. Each group insists that they have the one and only truth, yet they never seem capable of convincing other groups of the errors of their ways.

Because of this endless divergence, I think we need to be extremely wary about swallowing a particular set of religious beliefs. At the same time, we cannot ignore the phenomenon of religion as a whole. Humanity seems to insist that there is something going on here that is not yet explained by science, even if they can't agree on what it is, and we should not take this lightly.

So let's keep these fundamental attitudes towards science and religion in mind as we continue our exploration of the possibility of physical immortality.

Chapter 16

Physics

Matter

WHAT SCIENCE SEEMS TO KNOW THE MOST ABOUT, having studied it for the longest, is matter. According to science, matter is something that has mass (weight), and exists as a solid, liquid or gas. Matter happens to be something relatively easy for most people to understand, because we can easily perceive it with our senses. We can see it, feel it, smell it and taste it. We have a lot of experience with it, at least at our normal level of perception, and at this level it offers few mysteries.

Energy

If the universe were composed of nothing but matter, then it wouldn't be very interesting. Everything would just sit there. Luckily for us, there is something called energy. Science defines energy as the capacity to do work. By work, we generally mean doing something to matter: moving it, or causing it to move at a different speed or in a different direction.

Energy is a little harder to understand than matter, because we can't perceive it directly. Potential energy cannot be perceived at all. You can't tell by looking at a battery, for example, whether it is dead or still fully charged. What we can perceive, though, is the work done by energy: We can see the flashlight come on, hear the engine running, feel the river rushing down the hill.

A few interesting facts about energy are worth noting. Einstein discovered that matter and energy are equivalent. That is, matter can be converted to energy, and energy can be converted to matter. This equivalence took so long to discover because it takes a very small amount of matter to produce a whole lot of energy. This is why, in day-to-day uses of energy, we don't usually notice the decreased amount of matter resulting from the conversion to energy. The formula stating this equivalence is the famous "$E = mc^2$." What this formula means is that the amount of energy released equals the amount of converted mass (weight) times the square of the speed of light. Since the speed of light is a large number (186,282 miles per second), its square is an even larger number. This means that the amount of resulting energy is enormous, compared to the amount of matter input to the process.

Another useful fact is that energy and matter are conserved. One can be converted to the other, and energy and matter can be converted to different forms (solids, liquids and gases, as examples), but nothing is ever lost or created in these transactions. If you carefully count up all the energy and the matter you have after an event, then it always equals the total amount of matter/energy you started with.

Entropy

One last thing to note about matter and energy is that they tend towards entropy. Another way of saying this is that things tend to go from an orderly state to a disorderly state. This is called the second law of thermodynamics. By "order," we mean some sort of organization imposed from outside the system. By "disorder," then, we mean the state of equilibrium towards which the components of the system will tend, if left on their own. By "equilibrium," we mean a stable state in which opposing forces are equally balanced.

Here is a simple example. If you heat the water on one side of a fish tank, and then leave the tank alone, you will come back later to find that both sides are now a uniform temperature. At the beginning of this experiment, there was some order imposed from outside the system: one side was hotter than the other. At the end of the experiment, the water had reached equilibrium, meaning that there was less order: both sides were of the same temperature.

Another way of looking at this law is to say that things tend towards a state of inert uniformity. "Inert uniformity" is another way of describing a state of equilibrium.

Some people think that the second law of thermodynamics implies that death is inevitable. After all, the only way a living being can achieve a state of inert uniformity is by dying. This law seems to dictate that all physical things must eventually wear out and run down. Why should people be any different?

It is easy to see the fallacy in this thinking by reminding ourselves that living things are *not* consistently worn down. The early days, months and years of a new organism's life are marked by incredible growth. During this period, the organism is not being worn down but being built up. What's more, advanced organisms such as humans can regenerate and repair themselves. We are *not* like inanimate objects, then, and so there is no reason why we need be subject to the same inevitable decay and decline.

To put this argument in more scientific terms, the second law of thermodynamics states that the entropy of the universe, or of any other closed system, tends to a maximum. It is a mistake, though, to apply this law to living organisms. The second law of thermodynamics applies *only* to closed systems. Any form of life is, by definition, an open system. There is no reason, then, to think that living organisms must inevitably progress from order to disorder.

Determinism

Scientists once believed pretty strongly in a completely deterministic universe. That is, they believed that all future actions could be completely predetermined, if we could only accurately measure the current size, location and speed of all particles at a particular point in time.

In our normal inanimate environment, this seems like a pretty reasonable notion. After all, scientists and engineers have been able to accomplish all of their modern marvels only by being able to predict with great certainty what complex inanimate objects will do.

If you don't believe in determinism, then consider the timing belt on my car. The manual said to change it at 60,000 miles. At 60,104 miles, just two days before my appointment with the mechanic, the belt dutifully broke and left me stranded beside the freeway. If humans can build a device that will fail with such precision, then you have to admit there is a pretty strong case for determinism!

In a completely deterministic universe, of course, free will could have no place. All our thoughts and actions would have been determined long ago at some starting point. This view naturally gives rise to thoughts of a God, since there must have been some force that initially set the whole complicated contraption in motion.

Modern physics, though, has found limits to determinism. Forecasters once viewed the weather as a deterministic system. As supercomputers grew larger, they began to have hopes that they could more accurately predict the weather. It turned out, though, that greater computing power made no difference – it still rained on people's well-planned picnics. This observation gave rise to a whole new way for science to look at certain classes of systems. These sorts of systems had previously been dismissed by scientists as only turbulent, or random in nature. A new theory began to evolve to describe these systems: chaos theory was born.

Chaos theory asserts that, in certain types of systems, very small differences in the starting conditions can have enormous impacts on later events. Edward Lorenz, the meteorologist from MIT who first applied chaos theory to weather patterns, dubbed this the "butterfly effect." He called it this because of the possibility that the flapping of a pair of butterfly wings in South America could later give rise to a tornado in Texas.

Another challenge to determinism has come at the subatomic level. Scientists have verified that there are absolute limits to the certainty with which we can measure particles, as they get increasingly small. What they have realized is that there is no way to measure the position or speed of a particle without at the same time changing its position or speed. In our normal macroscopic world, this influence is too small to be noticeable, and so is barely significant. When we get down to the smallest particles that make up all matter, though, we find that this influence is substantial.

This effect is called Heisenberg's uncertainty principle. Determinism, then, falls apart at this subatomic level because precise measurement is fundamentally impossible. No matter how good our instruments, there is information at this level that is fundamentally unknowable, which in turn means that the future behavior of these particles cannot be precisely determined. Exit determinism, stage right.

Quantum Reality

But the nature of subatomic reality gets even stranger. Because of the uncertainty principle, scientists cannot specify the exact location of a subatomic particle. Instead, all they can do is assign a range of probabilities to its possible locations. This sounds reasonable, but the same scientists go on to assert that the problem is not just that we don't know a particle's position. It is, rather, that these particles have no exact location, until they can be observed. Instead, they have a partial existence at all possible locations.

It is like trying to make a date with an indecisive friend. He may want to go to the movies, or he may want to go to a concert. He just can't decide. And though you can assign probabilities to each possible outcome, there is no way of knowing what his decision really is until you pin him down. It is not just that he hasn't revealed his decision to you: he hasn't even made it yet. And he won't make it until you pin him down. These sub-atomic particles are like this: they like to keep all their options open. As Werner Heisenberg said: "The path of the electron comes into existence only when we observe it."[29]

This view of reality has produced a famous paradox by the name of "Schrödinger's cat." It is named after Erwin Schrödinger, one of the founders of quantum mechanics, who first proposed this problem. Suppose that we put a cat inside a box, along with a device that will measure the location of a single electron. Then further suppose that the cat will be poisoned by this device if the electron is in one position, and left alive if the electron is somewhere else. We have already said that the electron has no definite location until it is observed.

So what does this mean about the cat? Is it alive or is it dead? Or, as some scientists have proposed, is it half-alive and half-dead? Or alive in one possible universe, and dead in a parallel one?

If all this sounds unlike any reality we are used to, it may be comforting to know that it seems just as strange to many of the physicists who have proven it to be true. As Niels Bohr remarked: "Those who are not shocked when they first come across quantum theory cannot possibly have understood it."[30] Erwin Schrödinger once exclaimed, "If I had known that one has to accept this damned quantum jump, I'd never have gotten involved with quantum mechanics."[31] And Stephen Hawking garnered many votes for sheriff when he said: "Every time I hear about Schrödinger's cat, I want to reach for my gun."[32]

Yet these are the same people who have irrefutably proven some of the most unsettling principles of quantum physics. It is not, then, that these views are crazy. It is rather, that reality at the subatomic level is much stranger than anyone could ever have predicted. At the core of this comfortable, everyday reality that we are familiar with, there lies this unpredictable subatomic realm.

Quantum Machines

Computer programmers often build elaborate security systems into their products, to prevent unauthorized access. At the same time, though, they often build in hidden "back doors": some secret way in that is known only to the author. In the case of chaos theory, and this subatomic unpredictability, it is as if Nature had left open a back door by which something unpredictable could sneak in.

If some mysterious force threw your beach ball in the ocean with no use of matter or energy, then this act would defy the laws of well-established science. It would be impossible, according to our best knowledge. Yet, if the same force were to push a few electrons around, then science would find no fault. Given our relatively new insight into the nature of subatomic reality, this sort of intervention would be possible.

Of course, nudging a few electrons here and there is not very interesting. But what if we could build a machine that would take these subatomic events and amplify them – much as in the case of Schrödinger's cat? What if we could build a machine that would allow these unpredictable happenings to operate at the subatomic level? And what, then, if this machine could magnify the effects of these happenings, making them manifest at our everyday level of reality? What would such a machine look like?

To answer this question, you need not go very far. Look in a mirror. You are such a machine.

Chapter 17

Biology

Life

As I said earlier, physics says that things tend towards a state of inert uniformity. The surface of the moon is a good example of this state. Not much going on there. Lots of matter. Lots of potential energy. Lots of energy visible from a distant sun. Other than that, though, not much happening.

The surface of our earth is a very different sort of place. Lots of movement. Lots of change. Lots of variety. Everything but inert uniformity. Yet it's the same matter. The same laws of energy. So what makes us so different?

Life. Our world is teeming with life, whereas the surface of the moon, as far as we've been able to tell, is completely lifeless. So right off the bat we have to make note that life makes a big difference.

And yet life is definitely full of matter and energy. All living organisms are composed of matter. All living organisms use energy to ceaselessly move that matter around: hearts pumping, legs running, lungs breathing.

So the big question is: what makes life so different?

Scientists are now fairly convinced that life has been around for at least three billion of planet earth's 4.6 billion years. Humans have been speculating about the nature of life for at least the last 3,000 years. Yet it has only been in about the last 100 years that the defining element of life has been identified.

The defining element of life is evolution, as described by Charles Darwin in his book *On the Origin of Species,* first published in 1859. As A.G. Cairns-Smith says, in searching for a suitable definition, "life is a product of evolution."[33]

Evolution

Life, then, is all about evolution. Let's take a look, then, at the basic mechanisms of this process.

> 1. **Organisms.** An organism is something with organization, with structure, with cohesion, and with some distinct identity separate from that of its environment.
>
> 2. **Reproduction.** These organisms have to be able to replicate themselves. The replicas they produce should not be perfect copies, but they must share a certain number of common traits. These replicas must also be new organisms that are themselves capable of participation in the mechanisms of evolution.
>
> 3. **Competition.** Similar organisms must compete with each other in such a way that the winners of the competition will have more chances to reproduce than the losers.
>
> 4. **Variation.** The reproductive process should not produce perfect copies, but instead must produce some level of variation between parents and offspring. These variations, of course, will confer advantages or disadvantages

within the competition just described. Further, these variations must be capable of themselves being passed on to subsequent generations.

Although evolution is a relatively new theory, and has generated much controversy, it is by now well accepted in the scientific community. In fact, modern biology is pretty much unthinkable without the theory of evolution. The theory meshes with so many observations that it is impossible to extricate it from the rest of this branch of science. A.G. Cairns-Smith puts it like this.

> The idea that the multitudinous forms of life on the earth have evolved from common ancestors owes its security not to some single demonstration but to a more day-to-day experience of biologists – that this idea fits with innumerable detailed and general observations.[34]

In other words, even though evolution is a relatively recent development, because it has come to explain so much that was otherwise mysterious, this theory is now inseparably woven into the modern science of biology.

One of the interesting things to note about evolution is that it is an inherently creative process. New life forms evolve from older ones. Larger and more complex life forms have evolved from smaller and simpler ones. This ongoing act of creation is an inherent part of the process. It does not require some puppet master in the background pulling the strings. Once the necessary starting conditions are available, then evolution just "happens," without needing to be guided or directed by any external intelligence.

Life and Death

Given this background in biology, let's now take a look at the phenomenon of death, and see how it fits in.

Most people accept death as a fact of life. They see it as a given, as a biological necessity, as a natural consequence of birth. After all, aging and death seem to be universal traits evident in all the myriad life forms on our planet.

Is death really a necessary part of life, though? To answer this question, we must distinguish between two different sources of death.

Death From Without

The first set of sources can be said to be external. They come from somewhere outside the organism. Looking at the description of evolution given above, we can see that this sort of death is almost required to make evolution function properly. We said that one component of evolution was competition. The demands of evolution could be satisfied, strictly speaking, by simply denying reproductive rights to the loser. This happens anyway, as part of the process of selecting breeding partners. It would be messy, though, to have the losers moping about interminably. It is much neater to kill them off at some point, and clear the playing field.

The other relevant form of competition, though, is based on the simple ability of the organism to survive until it can reproduce. For this type of competition to work, something must be waiting to kill off the losers: predators, nasty weather, or a shortage of food, to name a few external sources of death. From this perspective, then, death that comes from external sources can be seen as a necessary evolutionary mechanism.

It is important to note, though, that the human race is already attempting to eliminate these sources of death. In what we loosely refer to as "civilization," we no longer expect to see members of our society starve to death, or to be denied the warmth and comforts of a family. So some members of our human species have already decided that this sort of death is no longer acceptable.

Death From Within

The other source of death is internal, through the deterioration that often accompanies aging. Once again, it is instructive to see how this process figures in the process of evolution. In this case, we can see that this sort of degeneration is a convenience, but not a necessity. Nowhere in the evolutionary scheme is there a requirement that one generation must die after giving birth to the next. Individual members of a species must compete with one another, but there is no fundamental reason why multiple generations cannot participate in this competition simultaneously.

Again, though, we can see that it is neater to clear the playing field between generations. This prevents messy interactions between parents and children, in the area of reproduction, as well as that of competition. It also eliminates "unfair" advantages of the older generation, due to factors such as their greater experience, rather than inherently better genes.

We can see, then, that gradual deterioration can serve as an important, although not vital, mechanism in the process of evolution. But what is it that causes this deterioration?

Programmed Aging

There are many theories about why living organisms age and die. Some of these theories are conflicting, and scientists have not yet reached a clear consensus on these explanations. What is significant, though, is that none of these theories include any absolute reason why life must invariably come to an end.

Some of what we have learned about "programmed aging," as it is called, seems in fact to indicate that this process is somewhat arbitrary, and susceptible to enormous variation.

Scientists have learned, for example, that there seems to be a limit to the number of times that a cell can reproduce within a living organism. This would seem to place an absolute limit on the life of the organism itself. Yet scientists have also found that some "abnormal" human cells have the capacity to reproduce and function indefinitely. Although some of the examples of such "immortal" cells are cancer cells, there seems to be no scientific reason why the immortality of these cells is inextricably linked to their destructive capacity.

Many plants provide dramatic examples of programmed aging. The century plant, for example, grows for decades before producing flowers and fruit, and then quickly dies. In the animal kingdom, fish such as salmon also seem to age suddenly, again usually following reproduction.

Other animals show no signs of aging, and appear capable of living indefinitely. Examples include such aquatic species as lobsters, sturgeons, sharks, alligators, the Galapagos tortoise, and the female (but not the male) flounder. In all of these examples, the lack of aging is associated with unending physical growth, and the lack of any maximum size. At some point, the unusual girth of these giants among fish must begin to work against them, since immortals in these species would be easy to spot, and have not been reported.

Somewhere between these extremes – sudden death on the one hand, and unending growth on the other – are other interesting variations. For example, there are insect species in which a queen can live as long as 27 years, while other members of its colony have life spans measured in months. There is no genetic difference between the queen and the rest of the colony – the queen is simply fed differently, on royal jelly.

Again, this information seems to offer powerful evidence that the speed of aging is somewhat arbitrary, and can be influenced by a multitude of factors.

Accidents

Scientists are quick to point out that the statistical probability of accidents would eventually weed out all members of a generation, even if they did not die from other causes. This is usually the last line of defense for people struggling to find some scientific basis for a disbelief in immortality. After they have finally conceded that there is no other explanation for why we have to die, they conclude that it really doesn't make any difference. After all, they say, the statistical probability of accidental death will eventually catch up with us anyway.

I don't really buy this. I don't believe there has ever been a death certificate issued that listed the cause as "statistics." I have never seen anyone felled by probability. It usually takes something much more solid to kill someone off.

If you pay close attention to these sorts of arguments, you will also notice a subtle sleight of hand being practiced. People and animals are usually lumped together as statistical victims, and accidents and predation are grouped together in terms of causes. (Predation, by the way, is the scientific term for "being eaten by something larger than you.")

In actual practice, though, these two groups are quite distinct. Being eaten by predators is becoming increasingly rare among humans. We have won the evolutionary contest for the survival of the fittest. We have banished our rivals to zoos and game preserves, and we generally sleep securely at night, without having to keep one eye open for large game roaming near.

Wild animals, on the other hand, seem relatively immune to accidents. When was the last time you saw an incident on the evening news of a hippo being run off the road by a speeding cheetah? Either it doesn't happen much, or our news media are falling down on their jobs.

The truth is that most accidents are man-made, and that what we have created we can dismantle. When we make human life our top priority, then we will find ways to avoid situations that are likely to kill people.

The deeper truth, perhaps, is that most accidents are not quite so accidental. I have something to say about what happens to me: I am not an accident on my way to happen.

This assertion may sound unrealistic, but I have observed its truth on a personal level. When we see total numbers of deaths by various causes tallied up by statisticians, it is easy to believe that these people were just random victims of chance. When we see an accident reported by the media, all the focus is on the results of the accident, and little or nothing is presented on the events leading up to it. Again, it is easy to see the accident as a random event.

In the few cases where an accidental death has actually happened to someone I have known, though, it has been easier to see that the death was not so accidental. There were reasons why the "victim" needed a way out of a life in which he felt trapped. There were risks taken above and beyond those normally faced. My personal observation is that, in accidental deaths, there are usually several factors involved, often operating on multiple levels.

The bottom line is that accidents are caused by people, and can be prevented by them.

The Beginnings of Life

Some deterioration seems to be a genetically coded trait, like the color of our hair, or the numbers of our arms and legs, or the design of our internal organs. Aging and death, according to this theory, are features that are programmed into us by one or more of our genes, and are therefore susceptible to change.

Once one gets used to the idea of death being an option, it begins to seem like a quite highly evolved genetic trait. In other words, if death is not necessary, then it would appear quite unlikely that the earliest living organisms included the mechanisms of aging and death. In fact, assuming the situation of a few fledgling living cells beginning the job of populating an entire planet, the idea of a predetermined, limited life span for these organisms strikes one as positively bizarre. It seems much more plausible that our earliest evolutionary ancestors were not programmed to die, and that aging and death were only taken on later as evolutionary adaptations.

This vision of our earliest genetic beginnings would go a long way towards explaining the pervasive notion of some early Edenic state that occurs in so many religions. Many cultures include a belief in some past paradise in which life began. Judaic-Christian traditions, for example, would have us believe that human life started in the Garden of Eden.

The details of these stories, however, generally seem wholly incompatible with modern scientific theories that the earth, and simpler forms of life, existed for billions of years before the first human appeared. Scientists now believe that life as we know it began with single-celled organisms, formed from a chemical stew of organic molecules.

What would life have been like back then, at the very beginning? The resources necessary to sustain life must have been abundant, and competition for them almost non-existent. Reproduction occurred through cell duplication, so there was no sexual competition either. These conditions may have well seemed like paradise to our earliest ancestors, compared to later accommodations. So, as long as we are willing to picture Adam and Eve as single-celled organisms, we can adapt our view of the Garden of Eden to fit the latest scientific theories.

The Diversity of Life

Our world would be a very different place if all forms of life were independent of each other, and depended only on inanimate materials for the conditions necessary for their existence. In such a world, all forms of life would be very similar, and very simple.

Such a scenario is hardly possible, though. Evolution provides a means for species to adapt to changing conditions in their environment. New forms of life, and their byproducts, in turn become parts of those changing conditions. So it is inevitable that different species will evolve into interdependent relationships with one another.

This interdependence has itself evolved into a delicate balance. Earth's atmosphere began its history with abundant amounts of carbon dioxide, and essentially no oxygen. The earliest forms of life on our planet took in carbon dioxide, and gave off oxygen. As these life forms grew, this process of photosynthesis began to generate significant levels of oxygen in our atmosphere. New forms of life then evolved that used this oxygen, and gave off carbon dioxide.

Everywhere we look, we see the same sort of complex interdependence between living things. These interactions between the species are often as complex and varied as the interplay of cells within each organism. So what evolved were not a number of different species in isolation from one another, but a living system in which each species played a part in the greater whole.

Popular notions of evolution often focus on the survival of the fittest, as the dominant paradigm embodied within Darwin's theory. Nature is then portrayed as "red in tooth and claw,"[35] a savage place characterized by ceaseless competition between the species, as well as within them.

It is well to be aware of the practically infinite varieties of life on our planet. Look at all the variations in species – birds, insects, mammals, reptiles, fish, whales, bats, spiders, caterpillars, ostriches, elephants, and all the innumerable others! Along with the survival of the fittest within species, we must remember that another ruling principle of life is the survival of the different, the distinct, and the unique! Life thrives on diversity!

At times, it almost seems as if the entire world were truly a single living organism, with species acting as organs, and individual organisms acting as cells. This view is sometimes known as the "Gaia Hypothesis."[36]

The Human Animal

In ages past, humanity viewed itself as something apart from the animal kingdom, uniquely possessing a soul. Modern science has made it increasingly difficult to defend this position. Try as we might, it is hard to find any human attributes that are uniquely ours. Our traits may differ from those of other species in degree, but seemingly not in kind.

Biologists place *Homo sapiens* in the primate family. The more scientists study our closest relatives, the more they seem to look like us. Geneticists have determined that "99.6% identity is found between human and chimp ... at the level of the working genes."[37] The same authors go on to point out the following.

> On the basis of all the evidence, the closest relative of the human proves to be the chimp. The closest relative of the chimp is the human. Not orangs, but people. Us. Chimps and humans are nearer kin than are chimps and gorillas or any other kinds of ape not of the same species.[38]

Based on behavior, rather than genetics, a similar likeness becomes apparent. Recent studies of non-human primate behavior have revealed many similarities between us and our genetic cousins. Other primates form communities, bond permanently with their mates, fashion and use tools, communicate through language, and apparently feel emotions. No matter where we turn, abilities once thought uniquely human seem to be increasingly common throughout our family tree. The conclusion of authors Carl Sagan and Ann Druyan is that we are "deluxe model apes."

Even those who feel most strongly about the uniqueness of humans must admit that our species has frequently demonstrated its animal nature. Images of bestiality and savagery are not hard to find. But one need look no farther than the average corporation to find daily examples of dominance and submission similar to those observed in groups of chimpanzees.

It seems clear, then, that human beings are part of the natural universe, and not separate from it. We are made of matter and energy. We have evolved over vast amounts of time from simpler life forms, and before that from inanimate materials. We are part of the animal kingdom. We may have advanced to the head of the class, but we have not graduated.

Chapter 18

Our Human Nature

The Human Enigma

CONCEDE, THEN, THAT WE HUMAN BEINGS are part of the natural world and part of the animal kingdom. We may be at the top of the food chain, but we are still part of it.

This still leaves the question of why we are so different. No matter what our genetic makeup may be, we still look and – perhaps more importantly – act very differently than other primates. We may be only a "deluxe model ape," but what is the nature of the accessories that make us the top of the line?

Computer Evolution

There is an interesting parallel between living beings and computers. It is possible for computers to be "hard wired." A computer can be dedicated to performing a certain task, and can have its essential nature completely built into it. The computers that control our heating and cooling systems in our houses, or turn our sprinkler systems on and off, or regulate the fuel and air mixtures in our cars, are examples of such systems.

Other examples of such computer systems are the dedicated word processors that used to be around a few short years ago. These systems had processing units, storage media and printers, and could be used for only one purpose: word processing. They worked fine. So why have they gone the way of the dinosaurs?

They were too rigid. They were good at performing their single task, but people got tired of buying computers that could do only one thing. Once people realized that the same processing units, storage devices and printers could be used for other purposes as well, they grew impatient with computers that were so inflexible.

What people bought instead, of course, were more general purpose computers. These systems came with very flexible hardware, that could be made to perform many different tasks by loading different software. The software was divided into different levels. At the bottom was the operating system, and on the most flexible computers even this most basic level could be easily upgraded or completely changed. At the next level came system extensions and utilities that could extend the basic capabilities of the hardware and operating system: software to play video clips, for example, or access powerful databases. At the highest level came application programs that interfaced directly with the users to perform useful functions: spreadsheet calculation, information retrieval, and yes, even word processing.

Human Hardware

If we now turn our attention towards living organisms, we can see that most species are like hard-wired computers. Their essential natures are an intrinsic part of their existence. They have fur, or feathers. They have feet, or fins. They thrive in warm climes, or in cold. They live in jungles, or in deserts. They eat plants, or they are meat-eaters. All of this is determined by their particular genetics, which is the "hard wiring" for living beings. Their appearance, capabilities and behavior are almost completely determined by their genetics, and so they are at the mercy of genetic evolution.

People, on the other hand, are like general purpose computers. Our hard wiring is flexible enough that we can adapt to many different environments. People live in the tropics and at the poles. We wear a loincloth, a suit or a parka as the situation demands. We fly through the air, walk or drive on the land, and swim in the sea.

Human Software

A naked human being is like a Pentium or Power PC whose hard drive has just been cleanly formatted: tremendous power, but totally dysfunctional without some sort of software.

The human equivalent of software is culture, in the broadest sense of that word. The definition of "culture" that expresses what I mean here is: "The totality of socially transmitted behavior patterns, arts, beliefs, institutions, and all other products of human work and thought."[39] Culture is the sum of all human knowledge, attitudes, beliefs, patterns of behavior, and artifacts. It includes such things as clothing, tools and language.

What makes *Homo sapiens* unique, even among the primates, is not that we have culture, but the great extent to which we are dependent on it. In this we are truly like modern general purpose computers. Our hardware is nice, but it is worth nothing without the software side of the equation. If we consider what makes us human, and what makes us valuable as humans, we see that most of that worth comes from our culture, and not from our innate natures.

We are also like computers in that our cultural components come in varying levels. Part of our culture consists of things we all need to get along in society: clothing, housing, transportation, language, knowledge of laws and customs. This basic level of culture is similar to the operating system level on computers. At a higher and more specialized level, we all have skills and experiences that make us different and unique. These attributes are like the unique collection of application software and data that may run on two different computers both sharing the same operating system. This level is also part of our culture, in that it is not what we were born with, but something that we picked up along the way.

Cultural Evolution

It is primarily culture that makes people in one part of the world different from people living somewhere else, and that makes one person different from another living in the same land. We speak different languages, we follow different customs, we eat different foods, we work together differently.

It is also culture, though, that forms the primary difference between us and our ancestors. If you compare modern Europeans to those living there one thousand years ago, you will not find any large genetic differences. Huge cultural differences would be immediately obvious, though: differences in language, in laws, in social customs, in ways of thinking and supporting oneself.

From an evolutionary perspective, this comparison produces an interesting insight: the importance of our cultural evolution has far outstripped that of our genetic evolution. Evolution is the means by which living organisms adapt themselves to changing environmental conditions. It is now our cultural evolution, and not our genetic evolution, that is serving that purpose.

Technological change often seems like the biggest component of our cultural progress. But consider also the evolution of our forms of government and commerce. Monarchy has given way to democracy in many parts of the world. Feudalism and communism have given way to capitalism.

It is our culture, and our reliance on cultural rather than genetic evolution, that has put humanity at the top of earth's food chain. Genetically, we are not the best equipped species for survival. Many other species are stronger, faster, and able to survive longer in harsher conditions. Our culture, though, has allowed us to extend our innate abilities. And our culture has proven able to evolve much faster than our genetics. Genetic evolution is a monumentally slow process that takes thousands of years to create significant changes. Cultural evolution, on the other hand, moves much faster. Look at the vast changes in human life that have come about in only the last two hundred years: the industrial revolution, new art forms such as jazz, and the beginnings of a global government.

Implications for Immortality

You may be wondering what all this has to do with physical immortality. Just this: whereas death is a necessary mechanism of genetic evolution, it is not necessary for cultural evolution. When a new version of your computer's operating system is released, you don't have to trash your old computer to take advantage of it. In most cases, you can still run the latest software on the same hardware you already own. In the same way, cultural innovations can be implemented on human beings who are already alive.

Yes, you may be thinking, but I still have to buy a new computer every three years. The new models are so much faster and more powerful than the old ones that I need them to run the latest software. Admittedly, this is where humans and computers diverge. But it is precisely because our computers are themselves cultural artifacts that they can be improved so rapidly. In the case of our human genetics, there is no way to change the design so quickly. Luckily for us, our genetic hardware does not seem to limit our ability to enhance our cultural software.

Cultural change happens so much faster than genetic change that genetic evolution has become essentially irrelevant for humanity. And if genetic evolution has become irrelevant, then so has death.

Individuality

I mentioned before that culture is part of what makes one individual different from another, as well as making one social group different from others. We are all unique combinations of capacities, skills, attitudes, beliefs and tendencies.

I also pointed out earlier that competition is a necessary part of evolution. One sort of competition goes on between species. For us humans, though, this sort of competition has become meaningless. We are the dominant species on the planet. We have no significant competitors.

The other sort of competition goes on between members of the same species. A given species will evolve, and even evolve into multiple new species, only through this basic mechanism of competition between its members. Darwin found birds living on different islands whose beaks had evolved into different sizes and shapes, to take advantage of different food supplies in the different environments. All the birds seemed to have evolved from a common species. Their beaks had changed because evolution had favored the survival of individual birds whose beaks had been shaped slightly differently than others.

A prerequisite for such competition, though, is the assumption that individual members of a species all serve the same function within the species, or one of a limited number of functions. In most species, males all serve the same function, as do females. In some insect species, there may be functional differentiation between queens and drones. In each case, though, there are a very limited number of functions, and all individuals within that class compete with each other, to determine which can best fulfill their common function. This sort of competition is a necessary component of genetic evolution.

When we look at modern human society, though, we find that this is another way in which we have outgrown the workings of genetic evolution. All males and females in a modern society do not serve the same functions. In the workplace, we have thousands of different job descriptions, all requiring different sets of skills and aptitudes. Even within a single job description, different assignments will require different traits and backgrounds. Outside the workplace, as friends, family members and citizens, we have still different functions that are performed best by different people.

This is another way in which humanity has become distinctly different from other forms of life on the planet. The process of cultural evolution has created societies that are utterly dependent on networks of interdependent individuals. This has effectively eliminated competition between members of our species (except in highly artificial environments such as professional sports and schools). We should no longer be focusing on making each member of our species the best he or she can be at a very limited set of functions (procreation and survival). Instead, the fate of our entire race has become totally dependent on the values of individuality and diversity within our species.

The evolution of the human race, then, has brought us to a point where death is not only unnecessary, but actually harmful. For if every member of our species is uniquely valuable, then every individual death is an irreplaceable and wasteful loss.

Humanity's Role on the Planet

I mentioned before the Gaia Hypothesis: the assertion that the planet is one huge living organism. In this view, individual species function much like organs in a smaller organism, and members of those species function much like cells.

Within the human organism, different types of cells have different life spans. Some are replaced in only a few months, while others last much longer.

Brain cells have the longest life span. They do not die of natural causes, and when they are killed they are not replaced. This is because, presumably, their unique function is to store information, to allow us to grow and expand through our experience. Unlike other cells, they could not serve their purpose were they to be replaced periodically. To fulfill their role within the organism, brain cells have to be essentially immortal. Each one is irreplaceable.

Turning back to the larger scale of our entire planet, we can see that humans may play a similar role for the earth. We may be the brain cells of the planet, already having displayed a specialized ability to grow and change through our ability to learn. We may uniquely allow the planet to learn from its experience. And in that view, each one of us becomes irreplaceable, and our immortality becomes essential to help us fulfill our role within the larger organism of Gaia.

Human Nature

To realize our potential as human beings, we must acknowledge that we are composed of two very different sides. In order to be whole, we must fully accept both of them.

A large part of who we are, as human beings, consists of patterns on top of patterns. Starting at the subatomic level, there are certain patterns to our existence that are shared by all things in the universe: the basic sub-atomic particles. At a higher level, there are other patterns that define the different elements, and different molecules made from those elements. At a higher level still, there is a cellular structure shared by all living organisms. Other patterns are shared genetically only among the vertebrates. Still others are only present in the primate family. Others are unique to our particular species. Others are a unique part of our individual genetic makeup. All of these patterns – ways in which our cells multiply and divide, the ways our organs work, the ways we procreate and reproduce – are stored in our genes.

Many other patterns, though, exist as part of our culture, and not part of our physical constitution. How we communicate, how we learn, how we relate to other members of our species – all of these patterns are embedded in what we call our culture.

Other patterns exist within individuals, in the form of personality traits, habitual actions, and personal beliefs.

It is important to realize that part of what makes these things "patterns" is their tendency towards recurrence. These patterns tend to repeat themselves. The most basic patterns are the most sturdy, and the most difficult to change. Higher levels, though, have their own forms of persistence. Like gyroscopes, our repeating personal and cultural patterns lend stability and structure to our lives. We may sometimes rashly wish that we could wake the next morning to find ourselves "a different person." The truth, though, is that life as we know it (and even as we can imagine it) would be impossible if we all did that every morning.

In the same way, and for the same reasons, our common culture often exhibits resistance to change. And while this resistance may prove frustrating at times, it is again what allows us to experience a cultural identity, and some measure of cultural stability.

It is essential to realize that all these patterns help define who we are. I sometimes hear people affirm that they are going to "drop all their patterns," meaning that they want to stop acting in some non-constructive but habitual fashion. Luckily for them, they are not able to achieve their stated objective – if they could, they would disappear faster than the Wicked Witch of the West when Dorothy dumped a pail of water on her. For without many layers of interlocking patterns, we would have no existence at all. In a sense, then, we are these patterns.

At the same time, though, we have evolved to the point at which we can consciously change and create many of these patterns. The entire "Self Help" movement can be seen as a means towards helping people change their personal patterns. The "New Age" movement can be seen as the first fumbling steps towards changing many of our shared cultural patterns. Although these patterns are often difficult to modify, we are beginning to prove that we can consciously change them.

Our human identity then, is two-sided. In one sense, we are a collection of recurring patterns. In another sense, we ourselves are the creators of those patterns.

At all times, then, we must remain conscious of our dual identity: as a collection of particular patterns, and as the creators of those patterns. To pretend that we are one or the other exclusively is to cripple ourselves. If we view ourselves solely as patterns, then we become rigid objects, and necessarily view the act of creation as going on somewhere outside ourselves. If we view ourselves solely as creators, then we become disembodied ghosts, mythical creatures of "pure essence." Both views are equally one-sided and distorted.

We are both creators and created.

Chapter 19

A Turning Point

Our Evolving Culture Crisis

WE HAVE SEEN THAT HUMANITY is greatly defined by its culture, and that culture is itself a product of its own sort of evolution.

In our modern society, cultural evolution has been driven by two primary forces: technology and capitalism. Our technological capabilities have been evolving so quickly that they have driven many other aspects of our culture. Television, for example, has had a huge impact on all aspects of modern culture, as it has become our primary medium for communication and entertainment.

The other driving force has been capitalism: the impulse to make money, and to amass wealth. Capitalism and socialism competed with each other on a global scale for many years. With the fall of the Soviet Union, however, capitalism seems to have emerged as the victor, proving itself better equipped to adapt to changing conditions in the global economic environment.

These two forces – technology and capitalism – can be seen to be dominant ones precisely because the conditions necessary for evolution have been allowed to exist in their respective fields. The scientific method allows different theories to compete strenuously in their predictive powers. Those that fail to compete successfully are mercilessly weeded out. Different products of technology compete with one another, primarily through the mechanisms of capitalism. Superior designs drive inferior ones from the marketplace, and spawn continually newer models.

The same conditions necessary for evolution can be found in the field of economics. In modern capitalistic societies, corporations are the competing organisms. They continually strive for improved competitive position, and ruthlessly drive their weaker opponents from the field of battle.

Evolution has proven to be an effective mechanism for progressive change in the fields of technology and economics. The unbridled impact of these two forces, however, has produced an unprecedented crisis in our cultural development. Many aspects of our culture have been adversely affected by the relentless evolution of these two forces. It is not that progress in these two fields has itself been bad, but that we have no other means for controlling the impact of these forces on other areas of our cultural life.

Evidence of this culture crisis can be seen in many aspects of our modern life. Almost every group in the world seems to be trying to hold on to its indigenous culture, against the eroding onslaught of technology and capitalism. With no other vehicles for controlling our cultural evolution, voters seem intent on holding politicians increasingly responsible for cultural issues. Candidates are chosen based on their adherence to, and defense of, "family values," even though our political institutions offer no means for dealing with such cultural issues. Members of our society turn to religions, with all their primitive superstitions and illogical beliefs, simply because they offer a way to cling to sets of values determined by something other than short-term economic utility.

Taken together, this collection of symptoms justifies an alarming diagnosis. Our collective culture is out of control. It is changing rapidly, in many ways for the worse. Traditional cultural institutions have not been able to withstand the allied forces of technology and economics. Some of the results are increasing drug use, increasing crime, environmental destruction, and increasing levels of personal frustration, depression and anxiety.

But there is worse news. Human culture is becoming increasingly homogenous. We have become, in Marshall McLuhan's words, a "global village."[40]

From an evolutionary perspective, this is a disastrous development. Evolution is a blind process. It creates progress only through a process of random variation, with failures weeded out by competition. It can be viewed as intelligent and purposeful over the long term only if we ignore all the failures, and look only at what finally emerges victorious. In the short term, evolution is much more likely to create interesting failures than startling new successes.

However, since we have created, in many respects, a single human culture, we can no longer afford failure! If we had multiple cultures, then we could afford to let evolution stumble blindly along, knowing that some of these cultures would fail miserably, but that other superior ones would eventually win out.

We have now put all our eggs in one basket, though. If it is true that technology and capitalism are succeeding in the short run, but also creating side-effects that will be disastrous in the longer run, then we cannot trust to survival of the fittest. If our single human culture proves to be a failure, then it will take all of us down with it.

We have allowed our culture to evolve naturally up to this point. We have considered only two alternatives: either accept our current culture as it is, or retreat to the past, defending traditional values. Neither approach is working. Traditional values are inevitably eroding, and modern culture is being blindly driven towards values based on greed, power and survival.

To find a way out of this dead end, we must consider a third alternative. We cannot cling helplessly to traditional values that will inevitably change. But neither can we afford to continue to let our culture evolve naturally. Instead, we must take the reins ourselves. We must create our own culture, with our only consideration being to consciously create a future that we want for ourselves.

At the Crossroads

Planet earth is now at a unique point in its 4.6 billion year history. We are at a cusp, a turning point, a crossroads.

For centuries, humanity has pondered the questions of where we have come from, and of who or what created us. Our species has created a variety of stories to explain our origins. We collectively imagined that we were created all at once, essentially as we are today, a mere few thousand years ago.

It turns out, though, that none of those creation stories were true. Instead, we slowly and continually evolved over a time scale of billions of years. If we heed the wisdom of modern biology, we must accept that we are the products of evolution. We were created, not by gods that looked like us, but by a mindless process. By dumb luck, if you will. We just happened.

What then, is the meaning of all of these stories we fabricated, all these gods that various cultures have seen as our creators? If we are honest with ourselves, then we must accept that these have simply been projections of our uniquely human nature. The gods are not out there, but in here. These innumerable myths are valuable and true when seen as reflections of our own nature, but meaningless when it comes to explaining or describing our external reality.

A Turning Point

After many years of ignorance and confusion, we now know how we got here. Evolution brought us to this point in history. Survival of the fittest, and all the rest. Evolution has been working tirelessly on this planet for over three billion years, and has finally produced a species that has become conscious of this process.

Two paths now stretch out in front of us. On one, we continue to be carried along by the mindless process of evolution. Since humanity has now reached a point at which we have circumvented and undermined many of the basic mechanisms of this process, this path is ultimately a dead end. If we continue to multiply mindlessly, without competition from other species, then we will undoubtedly evolve into our own worst enemy. Because, to continue along the path of evolution, we need enemies. Our human population will continue to grow beyond any point at which we can sustain even the minimum requirements for life, let alone any significant quality of life. If we do not make the quantum leap completely away from evolution, then this process will inexorably pull us back down into it. If we do not rise above our history, then we will be immersed once again in the endless struggle for survival.

The other path is one of conscious creation. We have imagined for millennia that someone else has been driving the bus. We know now that it has been stuck on a kind of auto-pilot – there has been no one behind the wheel. Until we knew the truth, we had no real choice except to continue to be swept along by evolution. We now, for the first time in the history of the planet, have a different choice. We can take the wheel. And we can chart our own course. There are no road maps, or even any roads – not even any destinations waiting ahead. To take this path, we must truly be willing to be pioneers, to explore, to blaze our own trails. We must be willing to decide, individually and collectively, where we want to go, and what we want our futures to look like.

We have imagined that our destiny was being guided by a wise intelligence that knew better than we where to go. We know now that our destiny was formed by a blind process of evolution. As unwise as we know we often are, we must now face the reality that there is no one better qualified to lead us farther down the road. There is no greater intelligence, no greater wisdom, no divine hand to guide us. We have only ourselves to rely on.

To take this second path, though, we must be willing to step out of our past, to shed it like the confining cocoon it has been. One life has brought us to this point. That life has included the evolutionary struggle for survival, and sets of superstitious belief systems that have been products of our cultural evolution. We must be willing to shed these completely, in order to grasp this opportunity to seat ourselves behind the wheel of our own destiny. If we take this path, then where we are going will not look much like where we have been. To get there, we must be willing to question all the assumptions that have formed the baggage of our cultural ancestry.

Including even the assumption of human mortality. For humanity has outgrown the need for death. If we can face this fact square in the face, then we have the basis for building something new, for taking humanity's next step, for seizing the reins of our own destiny. If we cannot accept the possibility of our own immortality, then we are still trapped in superstition and ignorance, and will be driven before the blind winds of evolution.

Part VII

Value Systems

Human value systems are a subject of utmost importance to the survival of our race. In this section, I'll explain how the idea of physical immortality can help us transform and unify these values.

Chapter 20. Prioritizing Our Values

We often say that human life is our highest priority, but when push comes to shove, how do our values really stack up? And how can physical immortality change the equation?

Chapter 21. Resolving Our Contradictions

We look at how we handle situations where our values conflict with each other, and how a commitment to human immortality can help resolve these conflicts.

Chapter 22. An American Tragedy

This stuff really matters! I offer an analysis of how conflicting values contributed to a tragic confrontation in Waco, Texas.

Chapter 20

Prioritizing Our Values

The Importance of Priorities

WE HUMANS OFTEN HAVE BEWILDERING SYSTEMS OF VALUES. We say that many different things are important to us. All of these individual values sound good in theory. In practice, though, they often contradict one another.

When some of our personal values conflict with one another, then we have to decide which values are most important to us. We have to know which values come first. To establish this precedence, we must essentially have a prioritized list of values. We humans don't like to admit that we are sometimes willing to sacrifice some of our values for others, though. So we don't often admit to ourselves – let alone one another – that these lists exist. Often, the only practical way to deduce the sequence of such a list is to observe someone's actions. By determining how they resolve such conflicts in real life, we can reveal their value priorities.

A good example comes from my experience working for a large corporation. Business executives are easy to pick on, of course, because their decisions often involve conflicts in values, and are often made publicly.

The president of our company had decided that he wanted to do something to let his employees know how much he valued them. Someone came up with the idea of holding a "Teammate Appreciation Day." The decision was then made to give every employee some small gift, some token of presidential appreciation.

When the great day came, with much fanfare, it turned out that the employee gifts were plastic license plate holders, emblazoned with the company name, and the slogan "We're Succeeding Worldwide!"

Much to the president's chagrin, the license plate holders were a huge flop. Employees reacted to them with derision. Some anonymous poet immortalized the gifts in a humorous and not very complimentary verse that was rapidly circulated throughout the company. Few of these plastic decorations ever ended up adorning employees' vehicles. Many more were pinned up in our cubicles, looking as out of place as most people felt they had been from the start.

What made the matter worse was that our chief executive and his staff could not really get a grip on why the program had backfired so abysmally. While it was true that the gifts were made of plastic, they were undeniably attractive, and available in two different color schemes. The graphic designer responsible for them couldn't understand where she had failed.

The truth, I think (although few people would have articulated it this way) was that the disaster was caused by a glaring and embarrassing conflict in values. Our president had said that his top priority, at least for this day, was to show appreciation for his "teammates." Yet, when it came time to put his money where his mouth was, he chose as a gift something that served the company more than its employees.

As a gift, his choice had all the charm and sincerity of the license plate holders "given away" by new car dealerships to buyers of their products, and proclaiming the source of their purchase. (And none of their practicality, by the way, since at least the dealerships install them for you.) No one buys such a product. No one wants such a product. No one needs such a product (your license plate stays attached to your car perfectly well without one). The only purpose of a license plate holder like this is to gain some free advertising for the company producing them. So, when it came time for our chief executive to show us how much we all meant to him, he picked something that none of us wanted. Instead he chose something that would provide a little public relations for the company.

A clearer message couldn't have been sent. On our president's prioritized list of values, the short-term success of the company obviously meant much more to him than the satisfaction or well being of any of us.

The Correlation Between Priority and Longevity

We human beings are fond of saying that human life is priceless. The acid test of our beliefs, though, lies in our actions. And frankly, our actions often indicate a different set of priorities. The truth is that we are often willing to sacrifice human life in deference to other things that we perceive to be more important.

If we look objectively at the priorities of our values, then we will find that the things we value most are those things we think will last the longest. This makes a lot of sense, of course. So, if we rate things according to their expected longevity, we will find that we have also created a prioritized list of normal human values.

Lasting Forever

God

Eternal Truths

Abstract principles, like justice or liberty

Land

The specifics may vary depending on the particular belief systems involved, but almost everyone puts one or more of the items from the list above at the top of their list of values.

Lasting More Than 100 Years

Works of Art

Nations

Families

Sports Records

Fortunes

Companies

Buildings

Although these things don't last forever, they do often last longer than their creators. Accordingly, people often devote their lives to the creation of such items. It is often said that people try to achieve a sort of "immortality" by having their names associated with such works.

People

Since individual human beings have tended to last about 100 years, they fall here in the priority list.

Lasting Less Than 50 Years

Automobiles

Home Appliances

Relationships

If you honestly look at the groups of items listed above, then you will probably find that your own list of values includes items from this list, in this same order. It's not really surprising. It's only natural for people to rank things according to how long they expect them to last. A Mercedes is given greater value than less expensive automobiles, in large part because the Mercedes is expected to last longer.

Once we understand these simple truths governing the prioritization of human values, a couple of implications become obvious. First, it becomes clear why people often don't act as if human life were all that important, even though they say that it is. If justice is more important than human life, then capital punishment makes sense. If liberty is more important than life, then martyrdom makes sense. If countries are more important than life, then war makes sense. We may say that all of these things are important to us, but when it comes time to choose, our choices make our priorities clear.

The second implication, of course, is this: If we really want to put people at the top of our priority list, then we had better start treating each other as if we were going to last forever.

Which, of course, is what physical immortality is all about.

No Higher Purpose

We humans have often had confusing sets of values. We have sometimes been misled by our sense of purpose. We continually ask ourselves why we are here, and what is the meaning of life. The answers we find to these questions often shape our scheme of values.

Many of us go through our daily lives without consciously thinking of our purpose. Yet most of us do have some deep sense of mission, or a lack thereof, that unconsciously guides our daily actions.

It is important, at this deepest level, to root out any false notions we have. As humans, we have evolved complex systems of ends and means, of activities and accomplishments. We perform activity A in order to accomplish goal B. But what is at the bottom of this scheme? What is the basic goal that drives the whole mechanism?

We need to realize, at a deep level, that there is no higher purpose than life. There is no god we are serving. There is no cosmic intelligence we are trying to manifest. There is no standard we are trying to live up to. There is no state of perfection we are trying to attain.

When we realize we have no higher purpose, then we will see that aliveness is not something to be used, but something to be exercised. We are not to use our aliveness as a means to accomplish some personal or corporate mission. Instead, we are to exercise our aliveness for its own sake – for *our* own sake. This is not to minimize or reduce what I am calling our aliveness to anything trivial. On the contrary, this aliveness is everything we are, all our hopes and dreams, all our feelings and desires, all we are as a member of the human race, and the family of life on this planet.

The value of human life should be our only absolute.

Everything else is negotiable.

Chapter 21

Resolving Our Contradictions

My description of the immortal life may sound familiar to you. You may think that the beliefs, attitudes, feelings and behaviors I am recommending have all been discussed before. Much of what I'm talking about may even seem so obvious that you consider it to be only common sense.

An experiment I studied as a freshman in college, in my "Introduction to Psychology" class, made a lasting impression on me. The researchers composed a list of statements, and then asked the subjects to indicate which of them were so obviously true that they could be called "common sense." Many of the statements were traditional sayings that were easily recognized.

A large number of the statements were rated as common sense by the subjects. What made such a strong impact on me, though, was the high percentage of these statements that were obviously inconsistent! It turned out that the same person had no problem identifying two different statements as both being common sense, even when the statements clearly contradicted each other!

This experiment indicates the seemingly boundless capacity of the human mind to embrace contradiction. Did the sun come up this morning? Yes, of course it did, just like it does every morning. And does the earth's rotation cause this phenomenon to happen? Of course it does – we all know that. But if it is the movement of the earth that causes the sun to appear every morning, while the sun remains relatively motionless, then what exactly do we mean when we say that the sun "comes up"? The words we commonly use contradict the reality we know to be true, yet we don't even notice this common contradiction once we get used to it.

It is true that much of what I am sharing with you in this book has been said before. Yet, at the same time, many other common statements just as surely contradict what I am telling you. So, when it comes time for action, which statement will you follow? It's kind of hard to tell, isn't it, when you hold contradictory beliefs?

What makes physical immortality so useful is its ability to remove many of these contradictions. Claiming physical immortality for humanity allows us to resolve these inconsistencies, and creates a sound basis for our actions.

Let's look at some examples.

Death as Loss versus Release

Traditional Belief 1: Murder and suicide are wrong.
Traditional Belief 2: After a person dies, he or she goes to a better place.
Confused Actions: Some disturbed people have actually killed themselves and their families based on religious beliefs in a wonderful afterlife. Less dramatically, many other people simply lead drab, humdrum lives, marking time until "God calls them home."

Immortal Resolution: There is no better place to go. We are already at home. Every human death is final, and thus an infinite loss.

Life versus Afterlife

Traditional Belief 1: It is up to us to build heaven on earth.
Traditional Belief 2: What happens here on earth is of little consequence, since our ultimate destination is with God.
Confused Actions: People worry little about the long range consequences of their actions. For example, despite the increasingly devastating effects of human overpopulation, people continue to have large families.
Probably the most public revelation of this attitude in recent memory was a statement of James Watt, who was then US Secretary of the Interior under President Ronald Reagan. Watt justified the pillaging of public lands on the grounds that it would make little difference, since there was so little time left "until the Lord comes."
Immortal Resolution: If heaven is to exist at all, it will only be because we build it here on earth.

Capital Punishment

Traditional Belief 1: It is wrong to kill another human being.
Traditional Belief 2: The only way to deter murderers is by capital punishment.
Confused Actions: What lessons do people learn from taking the lives of criminals? Whatever the criminal learns is obviously too late to do him or her much good. Others may learn that crime doesn't pay. Others learn not to get caught. Others learn that murder is justified in certain situations. Others learn that might makes right.

Immortal Resolution: If every human life is infinitely precious, then the only justification for taking a human life could be to *directly* prevent the deaths of others. Capital punishment is not necessary to achieve this end, since the criminal must already be apprehended and imprisoned in order for the death sentence to be carried out.

Master versus Pawn

Traditional Belief 1: Humanity is responsible for its own fate.
Traditional Belief 2: The universe is ruled by an omniscient and omnipotent creator.
Confused Actions: People assume that whatever happens "is all in God's plan." They become passive, leaving everything up to God. Or, they act selfishly, but justify their actions by claiming that since they happened, God must have wanted things that way.
Immortal Resolution: Every human being is responsible for his or her own actions, and all people can take actions that will positively or negatively affect themselves and those around them.

Value of Life versus Death

Traditional Belief 1: Human life is priceless.
Traditional Belief 2: It is noble to die for one's country, and for one's beliefs.
Confused Actions: People needlessly sacrifice themselves and others for a "higher purpose."
Immortal Resolution: Any and every individual human being is more important than any abstract principle, such as truth or patriotism. There is no higher purpose.

Sexual Pleasure versus Procreation

Traditional Belief 1: Sexuality is a wonderful part of being human.
Traditional Belief 2: Sexuality is only appropriate as a means of procreation within a traditional family unit.
Confused Actions: Discrimination against homosexuals; guilt and shame over sexual feelings that come up in "inappropriate" contexts; prohibitions on the use of contraceptives; genital mutilation.
Immortal Resolution: Sexuality can be enjoyed for its own sake, so long as we keep the following principles in mind.

- We should make people more important than the satisfaction of our sexual desires.

- Our sexuality should arise as an integrated part of our whole person.

Body versus Spirit

Traditional Belief 1: Human life is sacred.
Traditional Belief 2: The human body is merely a disposable vessel for the immortal soul.
Confused Actions: People do not care for their bodies. People are physically unkind and harmful to themselves and others, believing that what happens to the physical body is unimportant. People think they have to deny or deprive their bodies in order to nurture their spirit. People justify starvation and other forms of mass death on the grounds that these "spirits" needed to go through this experience to improve their karma.

Immortal Resolution: There is no existence of what we call "spirit" without flesh. It is not possible to have one without the other, or to assign one a higher value than the other. We need to act in ways that nurture both body and soul.

Individuality versus Conformity

Traditional Belief 1: It takes all kinds to make a world.
Traditional Belief 2: It's important to fit in with those in your family, your country, your religion and your workplace.
Confused Actions: Conformity; rebellion; separation between "us" and "them"; attacks against those who look or act differently; appreciation of individuality in "geniuses" who make some great contribution to humanity, but fear of individuality among "common folk."
Immortal Resolution: Every human being is valuable precisely because he is a unique individual. The differences between us enrich all our lives.

Self-Reliance versus Dependence

Traditional Belief 1: People who need people are the luckiest people in the world.
Traditional Belief 2: Dependence on others is a weakness, while independence and self-reliance are signs of healthy individuals.
Confused Actions: Abuse of others in the name of independence; guilt over feelings of dependence; unrealistic pursuit of happiness without any dependence on others.
Immortal Resolution: We are all dependent on many other human beings for our existence and our well-being. We need each other more than we have ever allowed ourselves to admit. At the same time, people are more important than relationships, and none of us need to remain locked into abusive or demeaning relationships.

Resolving our Duality

Until now, humans have had no firm basis for their value systems. These systems have evolved over time. Like all products of evolution, they were created through a combination of dumb luck and trial and error. They have been transmitted and perpetuated through myth, religion and politics. All of these values have succeeded at times, but many are contradictory, and not all of them work equally well today, or in all situations.

When value systems conflict, people have traditionally found no effective ways of resolving such discrepancies. This is one of the many reasons why war has been so prevalent among human beings. It's not a very efficient means of conflict resolution, but we have sadly had nothing better.

A belief in the possibility of human physical immortality now gives us – for the first time in history – a common bedrock for a universal system of human values. If we believe that people can and should last forever, then we can put the protection, nourishment, and fostering of every individual human life as our very top priority. Once we agree on this cornerstone, then we can use rational and passionate discussion to build on this foundation.

Chapter 22

An American Tragedy

THE AMERICAN MEDIA GAVE MUCH ATTENTION to the shocking blaze that took place in Waco, Texas in 1993. A 51-day standoff between US authorities and a small but heavily armed cult ended with a raging fire that consumed the cult's compound and most of its members. Earlier in the day, the government had used a tank to break through a wall of the compound, and to fill the area with tear gas. It appeared that the cult's leadership started the fire deliberately, using materials on hand for just that purpose, thereby fulfilling the group's apocalyptic visions.

All of this proved a field day for the popular media, of course. Cult experts appeared everywhere, providing professional explanations of the group's behavior, giving alarming estimates of the number of similar enclaves scattered across the American countryside, and hinting darkly at the possibility of more surprises awaiting us, perhaps in tomorrow's headlines.

Running through almost all of this commentary was the underlying, unspoken assumption that what happened in Waco was some inexplicable anomaly, some terribly alien intrusion onto our American landscape. The very existence of professionals who make their livings explaining cults affirms our belief in the strangeness of these people. It was as if their behavior were so far outside the normal realm that mere psychologists would not be up to the job – nothing less than a "cult expert" would do.

Like most people, I passively accepted this attitude, at least for the first few days after the conclusion to the siege. Then it occurred to me to wonder: exactly what it was about this group in Waco that made it seem so strange to us? The funny thing was – I couldn't think of any good answers.

Was it the violent nature of the conflict? Obviously not, since we see daily evidence of violence of every sort, reported by every form of our media.

Was it the fact that these people were armed to the teeth, and prepared to openly use their weapons against our government? But our US Constitution guarantees the right of every citizen to bear arms. And when our founding fathers added this clause to our Bill of Rights, I don't think they were worried about National Rifle Association members who wanted to go duck hunting on weekends. Instead, they wanted to ensure that we would be able to protect ourselves from an oppressive federal government with a large standing militia on their side.

Did these people seem so odd to us because they were followers of some peculiar religion? This hardly seems likely. After all, this country was largely founded by people coming to the New World to escape persecution for their unusual religious beliefs. Since our planet has become noticeably short on new worlds lately, we must suppose that Waco, Texas is now as good a place as any to set up camp.

Was it the mind control techniques practiced by the leader of the group, David Koresh, that seemed so foreign to us? Surely we are not so naive as to think that our more mainstream religions are above using practices that are similar, if a bit more restrained. Perhaps you should spend a little time watching your local religious channel on television, or listening to a similar broadcast on radio. But then, we don't need to confine ourselves to religion to find suitable comparisons. Just take a look at any good TV commercial. Let's face it – companies would be hard pressed to sell some of the products they do *without* some form of mind control.

Perhaps it was the terrible alienation of these cult members that struck us as so peculiar: their feelings of being so distant from fellow members of the human race. Yet we need look no farther than *our* attitudes towards *them* to see a similar example. It is difficult for the media to even refer to them as people, almost universally preferring terms like "cult members" or "followers."

Could it have been their isolation, their insulation from reality, that made them seem so curious? This would be unlikely, considering they came from a country in which, according to a recent poll, one in three adults do not know about the Holocaust, and one in five say it is possible that it never happened.

Was it, then, the apparent willingness of this group to commit mass suicide, that seemed to us so strange? Yet the one common strand, uniting all the various religions we are free to follow in this country, is the belief in some form of an afterlife that is superior to existence here on earth. It was only days after the blaze in Waco that I found myself listening to a popular "oldies" radio station playing Norman Greenbaum's big hit, "Spirit In The Sky." In case you've forgotten the lyrics, the singer asserts that, when they lay him to rest, he's going to go to the place that's the best.

Perhaps it never occurs to you or I to take a shortcut. But I suppose that, having been surrounded by armed federal agents for 51 days, seeing the barrel of a tank sticking through your house, and breathing tear gas, you might begin to consider it an attractive option. At such a time you might also remember one of our country's most famous rallying cries,

"Give me liberty or give me death!"[41] If you happened to be 33 years old, as was David Koresh on the day he died, then it might also occur to you, with support from a few of the world's major religions, that martyrdom is not entirely a bad thing.

I agree with many others that the conflagration at Waco was a terrible tragedy. Like others, I want to do everything I can to prevent this sort of thing from happening again. Unlike many, though, I don't think the problem can be solved by topical surgery – by cleaning up a few isolated cults living behind barricades. I think we have to go deeper. I think we have to be willing to examine the very core of our value systems, and decide what's really important to us. Then we need to build a new, consistent set of values in which this sort of thing can never even get started, much less come to the kind of terrible end that we witnessed in Waco.

Part VIII

Human Relationships

Life would be meaningless without other people in our lives. We'll see how the decision to live forever can improve the quality of our connections to others.

Chapter 23. Social Consequences

What would be the impact on society if people were to stop dying? A thorough analysis shows that the overall impact would be strongly positive.

Chapter 24. A New Togetherness

The mind-body connection has attracted increasing attention in recent years. But we've only scratched the surface of a greater connection – the one between people.

Chapter 25. Human Gravity – Falling Into One Another

There is an attraction between human beings that is altogether natural, but deeply suppressed.

Chapter 26. Social Structures

We need to further evolve our social structures, to provide more effective forms in which people can come together.

Chapter 27. Immortal Support Systems

There is a rhythm of aging. It is vital that we build support systems that provide a new rhythm, of endless life.

Chapter 28. Technology and the Human Web

We modern humans are often entranced by the latest technology, ignoring the underlying human values.

Chapter 23

Social Consequences

MANY PEOPLE HAVE THE MISTAKEN NOTION that physical immortality is somehow anti-social. They fear that widespread and dramatic life extension would undermine the foundations of civilized society. These are legitimate concerns, so let's look individually at the issues that people typically raise.

Greed and Self-Centeredness

Many people seem to think that a desire for physical immortality is selfish and self-centered. It is as if they believe that life is available in only limited quantities. Each person is entitled to only so much, according to this perspective. If one person takes more than their fair share, then they will be depriving someone else of theirs, or so the theory seems to go.

I don't believe that there is only a finite amount of life available. I don't think that I rob anyone else of their life by my living. Instead, I believe that my life adds to the lives of others, as theirs add to mine. The more that I live, the more that others around me can live.

My desire for unlimited life is not a selfish desire to live at the expense of others. It is a desire to complement the lives of others, and to continue to contribute to a greater whole.

Economic Effects

People often think that physical immortality would have disastrous consequences for our economy. The mistaken assumption here is that people will continue to retire at about the same age, even though they are remaining healthy and living longer. I don't believe that this will happen. Retirement is only valuable as the reward for putting up with a boring job for forty years. People who love their work don't retire from it, unless health concerns force them to.

If you truly plan to live forever, then you won't want to live a life of retirement. It would get boring. You would want to continue to make a contribution to society, and to express yourself in useful ways. You cannot live forever by retiring from life.

On the other hand, if you truly plan to work forever, then you won't put up with a boring job for long. Nor, for that matter, would you accept the prison of a single career. You would take frequent sabbaticals. You would change careers as your interests and talents evolve. You would do what you love, but you would not lose yourself in a job, no matter how interesting.

Given this scenario, immortality would be a boon for our economy. Let me explain why.

People in today's society tend to go through three distinct economic phases as they age. For approximately the first 20 years of their lives, they are an economic drain, requiring expensive education as well as other care. For the next 40 or so years, they are economic contributors. Then, for the last 10 – 20 years of their lives, they again become an economic drain, as they stop working and require increasingly expensive medical care. In other words, our economy today gets about four parts positive contribution compared to three parts drain.

Now let's see what will happen to this equation as human life spans increase. As an example, let's just consider the positive effects of people living to be 100, without becoming ill and dependent. By the time someone lives this long, they will rack up 80 years of positive contribution for only 20 years of drain. This increased return on our investment would tremendously strengthen our economy, not weaken it.

An additional bonus for society would be the continued development – and the ongoing contributions – of people who are leaders in their fields. Many people will tell you that it takes thirty to forty years to achieve mastery in a particular field. As it is now, these people have relatively few years available to work at the heights of their powers. The longer people live, the more they will be able to learn, and the greater will be their achievements. Can you imagine what Albert Einstein would have gone on to achieve, if he were still alive today?

Stagnation

Would society stagnate, if we didn't periodically kill off the older generation and replace it with something new?

It is true that, until now, it has sometimes seemed "hard to teach an old dog new tricks." Many beliefs, behaviors and cultural tastes, once rooted in a generation, seem difficult to change. It has been easier to wait for a new generation to come along, and try to make changes in people while they are still young, before their minds have hardened into rigid patterns. Cultural evolution has mimicked genetic evolution, and has seemed to require the birth of a new generation to make significant changes.

I do not deny any of this. But, if we are to live forever, then we must learn to become more fluid. We must welcome change. We must learn to evolve on our two feet. Each individual must be ever changing. Immortality would have no meaning if it simply meant the preservation of eternal stagnation.

Moreover, the acceptance of immortality causes us to become more fluid. When we set our sights on forever, we automatically give up rigidity. Once we begin looking forward to tomorrow, and to an endless series of tomorrows, then we can no longer hold on to yesterday.

When people live like this, then there is no "generation gap." People do not dress and act "their age." Each person, whatever his age, is a true individual.

Human Overpopulation

Population growth rates are dependent on two separate factors: birth rates and death rates. What's obvious is that immortality will decrease (or eliminate) death rates, thereby tending to increase the size of our human population.

What's not so obvious are the effects immortality has on birth rates. Even though human life spans have been on the rise, the biggest contributor to the growth in our population has been unrestrained birth rates. This is because many people have still been operating out of the old drive to ensure survival of our species through maximum reproduction. Another way to say this is that people have been attempting to achieve immortality through their children.

As people make the shift to physical immortality, they lose this drive to produce as many offspring as possible. Instead, many people are content to have only one or two children. Others prefer to have none themselves, even though they enjoy and spend time with children conceived by others.

I believe that these two effects – falling death rates and falling birth rates – will tend to balance each other out. Population levels may continue to grow, but they are already doing that. The net effect of immortality on population growth rates should be to keep them level or even decrease them.

Environmental Concerns

Will physical immortality make issues such as pollution even worse than they are today? I don't believe so. In fact, I am convinced that immortality will help increase our environmental responsibility.

Beliefs in the transience of human existence, and in the importance of an afterlife, have tended to make humans devalue our physical environment. We have been a bit like renters, who know that we will be moving on before long, and so don't really invest our time and energy in our current home.

Once we make the decision to live forever, though, we have new reason to preserve and improve our environment. We become owners. We lay claim to the world we inhabit, and so we consequently take better care of it.

For too long now we have said that we must preserve this world "for future generations." This motivation has not worked. We must begin to see ourselves here a hundred and a thousand years from now, and save the world for ourselves, as well as for others.

Acceptance of the principles of physical immortality, as outlined in this book, would also remove any religious illusions about it being humanity's "right" to breed uncontrollably and plunder our planet's limited natural resources.

Social Inequity

Another concern is that the availability of physical immortality for the well-to-do would increase disparities between the rich and the poor, creating a terrible ethical dilemma for society.

My first response is that moral dilemmas and divisions within humanity are already about as bad as they can get. We already have some people being pampered at spas while others starve. We already have people gunning down doctors in the name of a "right to life." We already have people killing each other over differences of race and religion. For a society in this condition, it seems a bit fastidious to worry about ethical dilemmas resulting from too much life. Perhaps we should first turn our attention to the ones caused by too much death.

My second response to this concern is that I think immortality will help reduce divisions in our society. I have already seen physical immortality make possible a world community in which Germans and Jews, Arabs and Israelis, and people from all walks of life and ethnic backgrounds meet regularly to celebrate their togetherness. If immortality can produce this effect, then I think we need to encourage it all we can.

My final response is that I do not think anyone who embraces immortality can be callous about people who are suffering due to social or economic inequities. To be immortal is to commit oneself to living with other people forever. This commitment can only result in efforts to make immortality available to all who choose it.

Moral Fiber

Some think that people are amoral, or actually evil, and need to be controlled to prevent them from being destructive. In this view, heaven is a necessary carrot, and hell an essential stick, to induce people to live in some degree of harmony. Without these two extremes, the theory goes, chaos would result. The increasing violence in our society, coupled with a corresponding decline in religious beliefs, seems to offer corroboration for this view.

I believe, on the other hand, that the increasing violence in our society is caused by the prevalent "death consciousness." People see the meanings of their lives as being negated by death. A belief in inevitable death robs our lives of meaning. So as traditional religious beliefs inevitably fade, people grow more cynical about the value of life.

With people committed to immortality, on the other hand, the meaning of our lives is clearly in other people. People naturally come first when you think life worth living forever, for yourself and others. And when we put people first, everything else falls into place easily.

In Summary

People who worry about the catastrophic effects of widespread immortality tend to focus on such problems as economic collapse, social stagnation, overpopulation, environmental disaster, social division and declining morals.

I could take these concerns more seriously if they were coming from a world where these problems seemed like remote worries, or where solutions for these problems were already well in hand.

Unfortunately, all these problems are already serious today, and seem to be getting worse. Immortality did not cause any of these problems. Yet people often assume that it will make all of them more serious – as if things would be OK, if only we would leave well enough alone, and not tamper with the existing order.

We need to do something drastic. I do not believe that we can solve humanity's problems by doing more of what we've always done. We need to try something new. Immortality has not caused any of our current problems, but it can help solve them – if only we will give it a chance.

Chapter 24

A New Togetherness

TRADITIONAL WESTERN MEDICINE has focused on corrective, rather than preventive, action. It has also focused on intervention through surgery and drugs. And while these techniques have been effective, we need to recognize their limits. When it comes to building health and wellness, as opposed to fixing problems, traditional medical science is just beginning to look at the possibilities. This is not a criticism. On the contrary, it is an exciting acknowledgment of how much work is left to be done. We have just barely begun to scratch the surface of techniques for increasing health and extending life.

The Mind-Body Connection

Leading edge doctors are now focusing on what is called the mind-body connection. This approach draws on the ability of the mind to influence the functioning of the body. Thoughts and emotions that originate in the mind are able to affect – for better or for worse – the physical condition of the body. Medical Doctors like Andrew Weil and Deepak Chopra have written eloquently about our abilities to heal ourselves.

We must recognize, though, how little science yet knows about this process. We know that some thoughts and emotions cause harm, while others do good. Yet there are infinite numbers of thoughts that we can think, and the subtleties of human emotions yield equal numbers of gradations and shadings. Are some of these more helpful than others? Of course. But does science yet know which are best? Can even the most advanced doctors prescribe thoughts the way others prescribe drugs? Not with any scientific certainty. And it is likely that such precise expert knowledge will not be available any time soon.

Oh what, then, can we base our decisions? Only on our individual and collective inner wisdom. We must trust that, at some level, we know what is best for ourselves. We may not always be in touch with this level, and we may sometimes have contradictory feelings, but we must learn to trust ourselves. There is no other way, no outside source of absolute knowledge that can guide us.

Most of this book is designed to stimulate your mind with helpful thoughts and emotions. So this entire book is working on the principle of the mind-body connection. Yet there is something more as well.

The People Connection

Scientists are also finding that the other people in our lives have a huge influence on our health and wellness. Research has shown that premature babies grow faster when they enjoy regular attention from caregivers. Other research has shown that adults live longer when they have a supportive social system.

Again science has established a connection, this time between human interaction and the functioning of the physical body. Again, though, there is vast variation in the beneficial variables, and no scientific knowledge to guide us. So once again, we must rely on our own inner knowing.

This connection between people is a vast untapped resource. The entire self-help industry is based on the idea of each person helping herself, and the mind-body connection is part of this. If our society has focused primarily on self-help, though, it is probably because we have learned to trust ourselves much more than other people. No man (or woman) is an island, however, and the influence we have on each other is at least as great as the influence we have on ourselves.

We take much of our normal human interaction for granted, but we must realize that most of it is constrained by our culture. Some cultures, for example, promote touching. Others discourage it. Our societies have very strict rules stating how people should interact with spouses, children, parents, friends and co-workers. And relationships that fall outside these narrowly defined boundaries are rarely found at all.

In some ways, humanity has made great strides during its relatively short history. We have learned the most about inanimate objects. We have learned a great deal about living organisms in general, and human beings in particular. In the field of human interaction, though, we have barely begun to scratch the surface.

Let's look at the same issue another way. Let's consider our ability to manipulate our environment to suit our needs. In the area of inanimate objects, we have demonstrated a great ability to engineer these objects to our satisfaction, building devices of tremendous complexity. In the area of living organisms, we have shown ourselves capable of selecting, breeding and training plants and animals to meet our needs. In the area of self-help, we have established the potential for increasing our health, wealth and happiness, as well as extending our life spans.

Progress in the area of human relations, though, has been so slow that few of us even think of this as a field in which progress is possible. Our current attitude toward human relations is similar to the equivalent attitudes about technology a thousand or so years ago. At that point, technological progress happened at such a tepid pace that few people were even aware of it. It has now accelerated to the point that we have come to expect constant change. Few of us yet think of human relations in this way, though.

Progress in the field is possible, however. Democracy is a wonderful invention, but it has taken thousands of years to implement it on a broad scale, and only the most short-sighted politicians would claim that we have perfected the institution. Capitalism is another feather in our cap, but it too needs work. Communism was an experiment in human relationships that has only recently been generally conceded to have failed.

Is much more progress possible in the field of human interaction? We might as well have asked a caveman about the potential for technological progress. It is only prudent, though, to assume that progress is possible, and to try to achieve further advances. Only by trying will we find our limits, if indeed there are any.

If we look broadly at human attitudes towards our fellow men and women, we can see three different categories of emotions. The first is repulsion. Before you tritely dismiss this feeling as inconsequential, we must honestly look at our long history of inhumanity towards each other. Indeed, we need look no farther than the headlines of today's newspaper to find fresh atrocities that people have perpetrated on each other. These sorts of daily attacks range from simple insults, up through personal violence and murder, all the way to genocide. So fear and loathing of one another is unfortunately an all too real element of human interaction.

The second broad category of our attitudes towards each other consists of simple disregard. To a great extent, we don't care about what is happening to anyone other than ourselves.

Apathy is another name for this attitude. As our modern mass media have vastly extended our knowledge of the human condition, without any sort of commensurate expansion of our feelings for one another, the size of this disregard has effectively grown. Our forebears had only their immediate neighbors to ignore, while we now have billions of people whose conditions we have to dismiss in order to get on with our own lives.

This may be a good opportunity to point out that our most advanced societies today are based primarily on these first two categories of feelings. To a great extent, our huge governments and complex codes of laws have been designed for the express purpose of preventing the abuse of one person by another. These devices have been somewhat effective. Even with the expenditure of such huge resources towards this end, though, a rising tide of crime is still one of our most troublesome social issues.

Capitalism is based primarily on the second category of feelings for one another, since "enlightened self-interest" is simply another name for disregard of our fellow man. Our governments have gone to great lengths to construct legal systems and economies in which our self-interest is aligned with the general good of society.

The third and final general category of feelings for one another is attraction. Broadly speaking, we could call this love, ranging all the way from sexual attraction to what some have called "brotherly love." These are the feelings that attract people to each other, that make us care about what happens to each other.

This last category has been a province reserved primarily for poets and dreamers. Marxism, as originally conceived, was intended to be based on these sorts of feelings, although in practice it never was. Utopians of all ages have dreamt of societies based on these feelings of attraction, of concern for one another. Christ spoke of such feelings. We all feel them at times, although we try not to rely on them, since they seem so untrustworthy.

Nourishing One Another

To build a nourishing human environment, then, we must minimize feelings of repulsion and apathy, and cultivate feelings of attraction. To put it another way, we must minimize human separation and maximize our interconnectedness.

How can we minimize fear of each other? One of the greatest human fears is the fear of abandonment. People are so totally dependent on one another, for love and affection, as well as for more prosaic needs, that simple isolation is as terrifying as bodily harm. This has become even more true in modern civilization, where violence is outlawed, but isolation is condoned and even encouraged.

Death, however, leaves all of us alone eventually. Knowledge and acceptance of our common mortality leave us with the certainty that we will eventually be abandoned by our loved ones, through their deaths or our own. Thus we all become afraid of eventual abandonment. It becomes, then, not a question of who will leave us, but when?

Even worse, this fear of abandonment becomes a self-fulfilling prophecy. For this fear causes us to shut down to one another, to armor ourselves, and to anesthetize ourselves in preparation for this coming pain. Separation begins, then, with the fear of separation, and grows accordingly.

The only way to end this downward spiral is through the assumption of immortality. Only in an immortal environment can we truly promise to never leave one another. Immortality allows us to create an upward spiral. By promising to never leave one another, we can end our fear of separation. And by ending this fear, we can create an intimacy between one another that will provide the nourishment we need in order to live forever.

An immortal environment, then, is dominated by human relationships based on attraction, rather than repulsion and neglect.

What would it be like to be surrounded by such feelings of attraction for one another? To feel love, instead of fear and apathy? Is there a way to nourish each other by cultivating these feelings? And is it possible that such nourishment could be part of a new human environment that would be more supportive of human life than anything that has previously existed? And could such a support system help extend human life, perhaps indefinitely?

We have no way of knowing except to try. Like the cavewoman fashioning her first wheel, we have no way of knowing where it will lead.

Chapter 25

Human Gravity – Falling Into One Another

Human Attraction

THERE IS A CHOICE THAT ALL OF US HAVE TO MAKE every day, and every second. It is a choice that is fundamental to who we are. I am talking about the moment-by-moment decision to allow ourselves to be attracted to other human beings, or to deny this attraction.

The attraction I am speaking of operates at a very fundamental level. It is not a theoretical love for our fellow man, but a palpable feeling of longing. It is not primarily a sexual attraction (it operates irrespective of gender), but it has this same earthy quality. It includes a desire for physical contact. It is easiest to recognize – because it is least suppressed – in our physical delight in the presence of children, and in children's innocent pleasure in human contact. But it operates at all ages. It is an attraction of aliveness to aliveness.

I say that the choice is "to allow ourselves to be attracted" because I do not believe that the attraction itself is an issue. To be attracted to other people seems to be a basic part of human nature. As humans, we play together, we work together, we make love together, all because of this attraction that constantly draws us towards each other. This is not a matter of choice.

What *is* at issue, though, is whether we allow ourselves to feel this attraction, or whether we find reasons to deny this feeling. This is the choice we have to make all the time. Do I allow myself to be attracted to you, or do I find a reason to get angry at you, to judge you, to fear you, to be repulsed by you?

This is what has kept people separate throughout the centuries: people have always let other things come between them (or have put them there). People have found reasons to scorn and despise each other, and to deny their feelings for one another. People have made everything else more important than human life: religion, politics, ethnic backgrounds, sexuality, art, ideals, science, truth and family, just to name a few.

This is the difference that we who have taken on physical immortality are making in the world. For the first time in history we are putting human life before anything and everything else that could come between us. We are putting life first! This sounds so simple, and yet it is completely revolutionary, and is fundamental to everything that we are. Without this feeling for other human beings, physical immortality is nothing more than a hollow theory.

This is the choice we have to make every day, and every moment. Do I put other people first, or do I let something else get in the way? Do I choose life consistently and continually? Do I exercise my choice daily? Is it an automatic response, or something I have to think about? These are the choices we get to make daily.

Ending Discrimination

Once we choose life, though, it is important to realize that there is another choice we do *not* get to make. We no longer get the choice to discriminate between human beings.
 I am not saying that we will be equally drawn to all people. What I have found, though, is that the degree to which I am drawn to others now is not so much *my* choice as it is *theirs*. Other people always have the choice of how much they are willing to be attracted to others, and to how much they are willing to open themselves up, to let themselves be attractive. Once I decide to let myself be attracted to human beings, then it is up to others around me to decide whether to open themselves up to this mutual attraction. I will be drawn most strongly to those who have opened themselves the most.
 To exercise one choice, then, we have to give up another. To choose other human beings means we can no longer choose to be attracted to people based on our own personal preferences or beliefs. We can no longer accept or deny other human bodies based on our own limitations. We cannot open ourselves up selectively. We have to open ourselves to all who are open to us, or we have to close down. There is no in-between.
 These are the differences I am calling for. First, we must be open to all human beings on the planet, without reservation, and without discrimination of any kind. Second, we must continually express the importance of this choice by our words, by our feelings, and by our actions. As immortals, we must choose to open ourselves to attract – and to be attracted to – other human beings, to a degree that is totally unprecedented in human history. By doing so, we will create an environment that will nourish human life as never before.

Let Nothing Come Between Us

So to be immortal, I must let nothing come between us.

I cannot let my ego come between us. I cannot let my fears come between us. I cannot let economic conditions come between us. I cannot let my independence come between us. I cannot let geography come between us. I cannot let jealousy come between us.

For me, this attraction to human life is as undeniable as gravity. This attraction of human bodies to each other is as basic as the attraction of planetary bodies, the attraction that causes one heavenly body to orbit about another.

Does the moon get to choose to whom it is attracted? The moon is attracted to the earth, and orbits around it. Yet the earth orbits around the sun, and the moon, of course, does as well. Can the earth and the moon decide that they will only be attracted to each other, and wander away from the sun? Can the moon decide that it will be attracted to the earth, but deny the pull towards the more distant sun?

For me, the answers are obvious. I have made my choice. I know the center of my universe. I am part of a human system revolving around a central sun. I am part of a global organic body with a beating heart.

People are the center of my universe. Living, breathing, feeling human beings. I am drawn to them as surely as the earth is drawn towards the sun.

And in our coming together, we become more than the sum of our parts. Together we form something new. We each retain our individuality and independence. Yet by acknowledging and accepting our mutual attraction, we can support and nourish each other as never before, and create a new human society in which people can flourish without end.

Chapter 26

Social Structures

THERE ARE MANY DIFFERENT STRUCTURES in which human beings can come together as social units. There are certain organizing principles on which these structures are based. Human togetherness in our society tends to function in the following modes:

- Through competition, by viewing other people as competitors for scarce resources;

- Through sex and family ties, for the propagation of the species, and of one's particular genetic line;

- In hierarchical structures, such as military organizations, governments and corporations, in which people occupy a certain spot in the "pecking order";

- Through sameness of cultural backgrounds, ethnic origins, religious affiliations, political beliefs, economic interests, or geographical locations, in which people group together because of some common trait;

- Through attraction or repulsion of opposites: liberals vs. conservatives, blacks vs. whites, men vs. women, believers vs. non-believers, etc.

None of these various ways in which people have come together have been totally nourishing. All of these ways of organizing people are reductive or destructive in different ways.

There is, though, another way to be together. It is an organic togetherness. It is the togetherness of the cells in a living organism. It is a togetherness based on unity and on differences. It is a recognition that we are one body, that we are the same in some essential way. It is this recognition of sameness that allows an organism's immune system to recognize all the different kinds of its cells as *self,* yet instantly recognize an outside cell as *non-self.*

At the same time, though, this immortal togetherness includes an appreciation of the uniqueness of each individual. This togetherness thrives on the stimulation offered by intense differences, just as a complex organism thrives on the variety of all the differing cells that make it up.

It is interesting to compare the evolution of human social structures to the evolution of living organisms.

In both cases, evolution towards higher complexity requires us to overcome strong forces that tend to pull us back into more primitive structures. The organization of a single living cell, for example, requires a number of highly complex and fragile organic molecules. Life as we know it would be impossible without such complex molecules. Yet, at the same time, there are forces at work that tend strongly to pull atoms into much simpler, and more stable structures. In order for life to evolve, then, it had to find ways to build and protect such complex molecules within the overall cellular structure.

Human society is similar. Forces such as competition and propagation of the species tend to pull us into very simple and stable social structures: lone individuals, and isolated family units. In order to create more highly evolved social structures, we need to be aware of these forces and take conscious steps to counteract them.

Modern society has grown dependent on relatively large and complex structures, including national governments, international businesses, and a global economy. Such structures have also proven to be highly unstable. When they collapse, the human cost is often huge.

To create a nourishing human environment, we need to continually evolve our social structures into more complex and productive forms, based on higher and more subtle organizing principles.

Chapter 27

Immortal Support Systems

I LISTENED ONCE TO AN AUDIO CASSETTE BY DEEPAK CHOPRA, on which he talked about entrainment. He described this as the process by which different entities come into rhythm with one another, when placed in close physical proximity. He gave an example of a baby placed on its mother's chest, whose heartbeat will soon fall into step with its mother's. Another example was of women living in the same household, whose menstrual cycles come into phase with each other. An even more interesting example was of identical pendulums that, although started at different times and in different rhythms, will synchronize with one another after a few hours. (It's reassuring to know that even inanimate objects succumb to peer pressure.)

There is a rhythm of life and death on this planet. Although its cycle is long and slow, measured in decades instead of seconds, hours or months, its beat is sure and measured. A friend of mine celebrated his fortieth birthday not too long ago. His co-workers decorated his cubicle in black. Then they gave him cards and presents gleefully informing him that the long, slow arc of his aliveness had reached its zenith, and was beginning its gradual descent into oblivion.

Scientists who once believed in a deterministic universe held that, if they could precisely measure the direction and velocity of all the particles in a closed system, they could predict with certainty the eventual destination of all these particles at any future point in time.

It occurred to me recently that, although Heisenberg's Uncertainty Principle has rendered such deterministic beliefs obsolete, something like the opposite truth very accurately describes human beings. That is, if you know the destination that a person has chosen, you can accurately predict their attitude (direction) and speed (velocity).

This truth becomes more important as, through declining birth rates and expanding life spans, the average human age increases. A large percentage of the human race now feels that they are past their prime, that they have peaked out, and that they are marking time as part of a gradual decline into certain death. They are no longer focused on their growth and expansion, but on their ultimate demise. No longer looking for the light at the end of the tunnel, they see only the dark tunnel at the end of the light. Their destination chosen, their attitude and speed changes accordingly.

Does this collective "over the hill" attitude have any effect on our daily lives? It's hard to say for sure, but I recently had the shocking realization that somewhere over the years my definitions of liberal and conservative have changed. I used to think that liberals looked towards the future, while conservatives revered the past. Now, I realized, the only difference is how far back they look: the conservatives to the fifties, and the liberals to the sixties. Neither camp seems to hold much hope for the future.

Would the world be a different place if all the people over forty were looking forward to hundreds more years of life? Or even if they just realized the *possibility* of living to 120? I think our choices do make a difference. It makes a difference to choose life. It makes a difference to hit 40, and set your sights on heightened goals for the next decade. It makes a difference to choose to support the aliveness of those around you. It makes a difference to be around people who are setting a new rhythm, a cadence of unending aliveness.

Chapter 28

Technology and the Human Web

Synthetic Interaction

I ATTENDED A SEMINAR SOME TIME AGO on the future of computing technology. The period being considered was the coming five years – a huge span of time for such a fast-moving field. The speaker described a number of trends, including multimedia and virtual reality (VR).

He described with great excitement some experiments in VR that were already being done. This work demonstrated that it was possible, even with relatively low-resolution devices, to create an illusion in which the participants could easily get swept up in the action. They would rapidly begin ignoring the telltale signs of artifice, and begin reacting as if the computer generated sensations were real.

All this sounded dazzling at first. As I continued to listen, though, I began to feel uneasy. It gradually began to seem that the purpose of all this tremendous technological effort was to create an increasingly realistic simulation of human interaction, when in fact there was none happening.

As the speaker continued to describe the wonders of this coming technology, it seemed increasingly perverse. Why, in a world teeming with humanity, do we need to spend such huge sums of money on simulating human contact?

The answer seemed to be that, since interaction with real human beings was so unpredictable and dissatisfying, we needed to create the means of programming something more to our tastes. Why endure all the annoying encumbrances of relationships with real people, when you can program a simulated human encounter the way you select a meal from a menu? Feeling frustrated with a co-worker? Just slay his proxy in a 3-D computer game.

Moral Number 1: Human interaction is so precious that we will spend millions of dollars trying to synthesize it.

Moral Number 2: Human interaction is so difficult and risky that we will spend untold resources to program it to our liking.

Back to Basics

Technological progress sometimes has to back up before it can move forward in a new direction. This sometimes happens as a result of different technologies interacting with each other in strange and unpredictable ways, almost like chemicals in a laboratory experiment. Until you mix them together, it's hard to tell whether the result will be an explosion, or simply an unpleasant odor.

A few years ago, desktop publishing seemed to forever alter the way we create documents. With the appearance of the GUI (graphical user interface), and the availability of inexpensive, high-resolution laser printers, a revolution took place. Suddenly the simple monospaced fonts of the typewriter seemed hopelessly inadequate. Varying type styles, sizes and fonts became a necessity, as did lines, boxes, shadings and the easy artwork of imported graphic images.

All of this technology still produced paper, however. Microprocessor-based computers were still considered personal, and the most common way of getting something out of your PC to share with someone else was to print a piece of paper.

Then along came computer networking. At first this was reserved for mainframe computers and their dumb terminals. Next came local area networks that could connect a small group of personal computers. Then there were larger networks interconnecting computers within a company or institution. Finally, there came the Internet, linking computers all over the world.

Suddenly paper didn't seem like such a good idea anymore. If everyone you want to communicate with has a networked computer, then there's no point in relying on paper, especially if some of those people are geographically distant. Sending them your document electronically is a lot easier.

At this point, two technologies clashed: desktop publishing and computer networking. The problem was that the recipient of your document could have different computer hardware, a different operating system, different word processing software, and different fonts. These varying system components could make it difficult, if not downright impossible, for someone else to view your carefully formatted document.

Technical resolutions to this conflict are possible, and are beginning to become available. Software vendors are now selling programs to create and read what they call portable documents: ones that can be moved to an entirely different computing system, and still be read with all their original fonts and formats.

A funny thing happened along the way, though. Technology took a different path. Electronic mail was born. E-mail software allows you to exchange notes with anyone you can reach through your network – even someone on a completely different computer system. And how did e-mail solve the problem of this technological Tower of Babel? The solution was easy – e-mail simply regressed back to a point before the introduction of all this fancy formatting.

That's right – when faced with a choice between universal electronic communication and elaborate document formatting, all the fancy fonts and styles went straight out the window. Without, I might add, much complaint being made or even notice being taken. Most e-mail simply transmits straight text, without even some of the features (such as underlining) commonly available on an instrument as primitive as a typewriter.

So what was really going on when people were saying how much their communications were enhanced by all these different typefaces? Why did it seem so important back then, and so dispensable now?

Moral Number 3: Human language, whatever the medium, is the most enduring and substantial form of communication: Never underestimate the power of the word.

Moral Number 4: In a world where other routes of discovery seem closed to most people, technology offers the adventure of exploring new territory. This exploration is personally rewarding for its own sake, even when it has to be justified in other ways at institutional and societal levels.

The Web

One of the features of the Internet attracting the most attention these days is the World Wide Web. The Web was the offspring of computer networking and yet another technology: hypertext. Hypertext consists of a bunch of words containing links from one point to another. Like hyperspace in science fiction, hypertext allows you to be "beamed up" (or around, or down). In both cases, you can travel directly from one point to another, without having to slog through the intervening territory a bit at a time.

Hypertext had been around for years, without generating much excitement in anyone except a small group of theorists predicting that it would be big someday. In theory, hypertext could free readers from the tyranny of linear logic, making the reader a navigator who could chart his own course through the written word. The problem was that hypertext, as a stand-alone technology, only allowed "jumps" within a single document. Since no matter how many times you jumped, you still ended up in the same place, it was not too exciting.

When hypertext was married to the Internet, however, the result was the World Wide Web. Using programs called Web browsers, you could now jump from the middle of your document to another computer site on the other side of the world. From there, you could jump to another spot, and yet another, perhaps never returning to your beginning point. These hypertext links could be created without the permission, or even the knowledge, of the authors of the destination documents. They could be added, changed, or deleted just as easily. The result was a complex "web" of interconnections that was constantly changing and evolving, and that literally spanned the globe.

What is the Web's source of appeal? It is growing at a fantastic rate, again representing a huge investment in new technology. And again, the reasons most commonly given are not necessarily the true ones.

Some critics have already pointed out that, despite the wealth of information available on the Web, much of the best stuff is still not there. One reason for this is that much of the Web consists of *metadata:* data about other data. With the right network address, for example, you can look up any book cataloged by the Library of Congress. If you want to actually *read* one of those books, though, you are out of luck: you'll still have to revert to good old-fashioned non-electronic means for that. Other realists have pointed out that, despite the number of businesses leaping on the Internet bandwagon, most of the evidence available indicates that such investments do not pay for themselves.

So what is the Web's true appeal? First, there is the adventure of exploring a new technology, both for the creators and the browsers of Web pages. Second, there is the joy of human interaction. Creators get to express themselves to a potentially global audience, and browsers get to experience these expressions from people all over the world. There is an excitement in jumping from one person's site to another. You can weave a non-linear thread spun from the choices you make and the paths laid down by others, creating a logic of its own as it grows. There is an excitement of interacting with people from all over the world, an excitement in the spontaneous co-creation of a togetherness that is unpredictable and ever growing.

Moral Number 5: The greatest exploration we have available is of one another. The primary role of communications technology should be to facilitate that exploration.

The Human Web

All these technological developments sometimes seem to mask the underlying and enduring value of contact with other human beings. We grow enchanted with the shiny new technology, forgetting that it is worthless without content, and that the content consists of living, breathing people. There is a person on the other end of the wire, and the primary value of the wire is the connection it provides with that person.

Is the person just as valuable without the wire? I was reminded of the answer in the summer of 1995, when I attended the annual convention ("Convergence," they called it) of an organization called People Forever. It was held that year in Herzlia, a resort town just north of Tel Aviv, in Israel. There were about three hundred people there. They were from Israel, and the US, from Australia and New Zealand, Venezuela and Argentina, England, Ireland, the Netherlands, Belgium and Germany. Most spoke at least some English, but some knew only Spanish.

Most of the Convergence consisted of meetings, and most of these meetings consisted of spontaneous expressions from the attendees. A microphone would be passed among the crowd. Each person would speak on some common topic – his appreciation of each person's uniqueness, her passion to live, his thrill at meeting people from so many nations, her desire to build a better world, or someone else's pleasure at feeling the touch of another human being. When one person was done, others would raise their hands, one of them would be selected, and the process would continue. One person would cry, another laugh, someone else would scream, yet another would sing, or read a poem. There was no prescribed topic. Someone would speak their heart, and then someone else from the other side of the world, and perhaps sitting twenty feet away, would be set on fire and would express their heart in turn. One expression. *Jump.* Another expression. *Jump.* Another, yet another. Weaving a global web, from one heart to another, following no prescribed path but only the inexplicable logic of the human soul.

Moral Number 6: We are one, and technology is a tool for exploring that oneness.

Jump.

Part IX

Religion

Almost all of us have been raised in one or more religious systems, and all of us have grown up in the shadow of religion. In Part IX, I'll explain how physical immortality takes humanity's belief in religion to its next evolutionary step.

Chapter 29. Physical Immortality: The Un-Religion

We'll look at the ways in which a belief in physical immortality constitutes a religion, and ways in which it differs from all other religious belief systems.

Chapter 30. God

The notion of God has been a unifying force in human affairs, and has been a powerful symbol for the harmony and order we feel underlying the apparent chaos of life around us. These feelings of unity are fragile and valuable, and need to be nourished and enhanced.

Chapter 31. The New Age

Many people today have abandoned traditional belief systems for what are called "New Age" beliefs. Living forever, as I describe it, includes some New Age beliefs but not others. So agelessness goes beyond the New Age, as well as old age.

Chapter 29

Physical Immortality: The Un-Religion

IS PHYSICAL IMMORTALITY A RELIGION? This is a tough question, because physical immortality embraces some traditional religious elements, but does away with others. As a result, some people think that physical immortality is too religious, while others seem to think it not religious enough.

For myself, I have come to think of physical immortality as the "Un-Religion." On one hand, its beliefs and practices are closer to a religion than to any other system of human thought. On the other hand, physical immortality is fundamentally different from every religion that has come before.

I believe that physical immortality is similar to other religions, in that it offers:

- a vision of heaven, and of how to reach this state;
- a belief in eternal life;
- trust in a higher power;

- a need for faith;

- an emphasis on spirit;

- an explanation of the nature of evil;

- a set of core values;

- a nurturing human community.

For me, though, physical immortality is different from traditional religions, in that it puts the responsibility for attaining all of these things squarely on human shoulders, rather than in the hands of some external deity. Immortality is also different in that it offers all of these things in the here and now, rather than in some far-off future state.

Heaven

All human beings seem to share some innate vision of the way things should be. The details may vary, but the overall outline of this ideal state remains remarkably consistent, from one person to the next, from one culture to another, from one era to a later one. Togetherness, harmony, peace, love, eternal life, union with a higher power – these are just a few attributes of an ideal condition that most people seem to desire, but that often seems impossible to obtain in our daily lives.

Once we realize that people share this common vision, then it is but a short step to the next realization: the function of religion is to explain the discrepancy between the way things are, and the way they should be. We all believe that life could be different and better. What religion collectively offers are explanations of why this disparity exists, and how it can be resolved.

These explanations differ widely. Some religions place this ideal human condition far back in the past, in an Edenic state. Others make it subject to some far off future dispensation. Some think this ideal state attainable through reincarnation. Certain religions see it as a state of consciousness that can be reached only by withdrawing from physical reality. Many claim it can be found in an afterlife, in the form of heaven. Some people believe that the streets of heaven will be paved with gold.

Physical immortality also serves a similar religious function. It too offers an explanation of this universally recognized discrepancy between the way things are, and the way they should be.

What is different about physical immortality, though, is that it offers this ideal state in the here and now! Heaven is not in some far off place that we have to wait to reach. The power to grant us access to this state is not in the hands of fate, or some mysterious deity: it is in our own hands. Physical immortality offers a vision of the world, and of humanity, in which heaven on earth is not only attainable – it has arrived!

For me, this difference is truly revolutionary. All other religions seem to be saying that I am just marking time here on earth – that I am constantly preparing for a better place, but never arriving. Other religions offer me rules, concepts and precepts that will supposedly lead to a better life in the hereafter, but that ignore or devalue my condition here on earth. In this sense, all other religions seem to be fundamentally disempowering. They place the ability to reach heaven in some realm that is never quite attainable by ordinary humans in the here and now.

Physical immortality, though, suggests that we can transform "the way things are" to "the way things should be" right now. Eternity, nirvana and paradise are only a heartbeat away, and the power to attain them is in our hands. This, to me, is the ultimate in human empowerment. We make the difference.

Eternal Life

All religions share a belief in some form of life everlasting. Death, although an apparently universal feature of human life, is obviously not part of the way things should be. Accordingly, all traditional religions include a belief that death is not final, but merely a transition to another plane of existence. For some, what comes after life is a heaven or hell; for others, it is another turn on the wheel of reincarnation; for still others, it may represent some sort of return to a spiritual source.

Physical immortality also says that life should not end with death. Unlike other religions, though, it does not try to explain away death. Instead, physical immortality acknowledges that death is real and final, but says that death should be avoided altogether.

Many people think that a belief in the possibility of human physical immortality is unrealistic. I do not see this as the primary difference between my beliefs and those of traditional religions. Instead, I see the following contrasts.

- Immortality is more realistic than an afterlife, in that it proposes to end death by simply extending something we already know to exist – life here on earth. Beliefs in an afterlife propose some new plane of existence for which there is no evidence.

- Immortality offers some realistic feedback about its possibility of attainment: you can see whether you are aging and deteriorating physically. Those who believe in a spiritual hereafter have no way of knowing if they are getting closer to their goal.

- Immortality is tougher to believe, in that it requires humanity to do something new to achieve it. Traditional religions offer the comforting belief that the path to an afterlife is already firmly established and well trod.

I am very skeptical about any sort of life after death. I prefer to put my faith in a reality that I can touch and feel – the reality of physical life on this planet. Further, a belief in an afterlife prevents people from investing completely in our physical life here with each other. This lack of investment in each other serves as an "exit to death." As long as we are waiting for a heaven after death, we will not create a heaven here on earth with each other.

A Higher Power

Belief in a higher power – in something greater than our individual selves – is a common element of all religions. Such a belief offers humans a purpose for living, and a reason for coming together to achieve something more satisfying than their isolated individual goals.

This higher power has traditionally taken the form of a god. In fact, many people would equate a belief in god with religion. What has distinguished one religion from another has been the nature of the god(s), not that you believed in one (or more).

As someone who has embraced physical immortality, I do not believe in a god, in the sense of some deity external to humanity.

Is it possible to have religion without god?

I not only think it possible, but that religion is better for it!

Although it does not offer a belief in god, physical immortality does still offer a belief in a higher power: it is something we humans create when we come together to support our common aliveness. There is something greater than me – it's you and me together. My trust is placed, not in a God, or in myself alone, but in a synergistic coming together of human individuals. As a lone identity, I am weak and fallible. There is much that I am not capable of. But together, the human community is able to achieve almost anything. So far, though, we have only scratched the surface of ways that we can work together to achieve this synergy.

As we come together to form a global body of human aliveness, we are becoming the higher power that humanity has always sought.

Faith

All religions include some beliefs that cannot be proved or disproved, but that simply need to be accepted on faith. Traditionally, such convictions include a belief in a god, and a belief in an afterlife.

Physical immortality also includes an element of faith. The most we can hope for from science, after all, is the admission that there is no absolute biological reason why we have to die. No matter how long we may live, it will never be long enough to prove that we can live forever. And even if we could prove a theoretical human potential for immortality, it will still require an act of faith to believe in one's own personal immortality.

By faith, though, I do not mean simply a passive acceptance of a possible reality. I do not require blind faith. The faith I am talking about is an active one. It is a deep belief stemming from a passionate feeling that this is the way life is meant to be, and that it is possible to have our hearts' desires.

Spirit

All religions seem to share a belief in the spiritual: in some force that elevates us beyond the purely material, and beyond the plane of mere animal existence. Religions generally also place value on the cultivation and evocation of spirit. Where religions differ is in their beliefs about the origin of spirit, and the mechanisms by which spirit animates flesh.

My belief in physical immortality is materialistic in the sense that I believe in nothing that exists apart from the physical universe. I do not deny the existence of spirit, though – I simply view spirit as a desirable, and variable, attribute of living organisms. In other words, spirit is still something good, and something to be cultivated. The only difference is that immortality defines spirit as having its source within living beings, instead of originating from some external entity.

Traditional religions often visualize spirit as something existing in a pure form that, when added to matter, creates life. In this view, our bodies become disposable vessels, valuable only because they temporarily contain spirit. Physical immortality, on the other hand, recognizes spirit as something that is an intrinsic, inseparable part of living flesh.

There is an aliveness that we feel, a quickening of the flesh, an anointing, an inspiration, an energy that flows between us: this, to me, is spirit. These spiritual feelings are wonderful, and it is wonderful to come together and inspire these feelings in one another. I have experienced these feelings when I have been by myself. I have felt them when I have been with other people. But I have never felt this sense of spirit emanating from anywhere other than living flesh.

People sometimes visualize a spiritual plane of existence that is superior to life here on earth, that is free of earthly constraints. I don't see things this way. I love being physical: being able to touch other people, to see them smile, to feel their warmth. I have it all here: spirit and flesh. I don't feel constrained by matter – I feel empowered by it. Even if a purely spiritual plane existed, why would I want to give up my existence here for some place where all I had was only part of what I have now?

The Nature of Evil

The second law of thermodynamics states that "the entropy of the universe tends to a maximum." Since entropy is a measure of the degree of disorder in a system, the implication is that things evolve from a state of relative order to one of disorder. In other words, things tend to disintegrate, to run down, and eventually to fall apart. If we are looking for an evil force at work in the universe, then I think we need look no further than the second law of thermodynamics.

Is there an opposing force? Yes – it is life itself. Life, including the force of evolution, tends toward states of greater order. A fully formed organism develops from a single cell. Life forms become increasingly complex over time. And these life forms, in turn, create other forms of complexity, such as tools, works of art, and other cultural artifacts.

My devil, in other words, is the second law of thermodynamics. And my god, in this sense, is life itself. In this context, physical immortality is a natural expression of life's tendency towards greater order.

Human beings are not inherently good or evil. Our actions can be destructive, or constructive. When we act destructively, it is because we have become separated from each other. If we fully feel our connection to others, then we also feel the impacts our actions have, and will naturally avoid actions with undesirable consequences.

Values and Morality

Most religions offer a set of core values that can be used to guide human conduct. Many religions also offer more specific moral codes, such as the Ten Commandments of the Christian Bible.

Many common moral elements are found in almost all the world's major religions. Many of these are wonderful values that help people live together in peace and harmony. Unfortunately, though, one of the elements most religions have in common is that the value placed on loyalty to a particular religion is greater than the value placed on human life. One of the Ten Commandments, for example, is "Thou shalt not kill." Before that, though, this Christian God says:

> Thou shalt have none other gods before me.
>
> Thou shalt not bow down thyself unto them [graven images], nor serve them: for I the Lord thy God am a jealous God….
>
> Thou shalt not take the name of the Lord thy God in vain….[42]

What happens, then, when the love of god seems to conflict with the love of people?

The results of this moral ambiguity, in terms of human suffering, have been devastating. Millions of people have been killed in the name of religion. Others have cut their own lives short, to satisfy their notion of a god, or to speed their arrival in heaven. Others have suffered while alive, in the belief that their hardships were ordained by god.

Despite this divided loyalty, many people still think that we nonetheless need a god to enforce moral standards. Many people believe that humans are basically amoral, or actually evil, and that we have no hope of living up to any moral standards without forceful direction from an almighty being. Without god, then, they believe there can be no morality.

The values associated with physical immortality do not have such a deity to back them up. I find, though, that these values spring naturally from my human nature, my desire to be part of human society, my feelings for other people, and my decision to stay here forever. After all, if I'm going to be here forever, then the consequences of my actions are bound to catch up with me eventually. So my morality does not suffer for lack of a god.

What, then, are these values?

Physical immortality is the first belief system to proclaim that people are more important than truth, that you are more important than any beliefs, and that our togetherness is more important than our intellectual agreement. Physical immortality, for the first time in human history, places an absolute value on human life. This leaves no excuse for separation on the grounds of religious differences.

Because those of us believing in physical immortality think that people are more important than truth, we do not have any stringent moral code set forth by a sacred text. What we do have is a feeling for each other that continues to grow the more we exercise it, and that guides our actions more surely and precisely than could any law.

Community

One of the things I have always appreciated most about organized religion is its ability to bring people together and create a sense of community. Churches of many denominations have served as centers for social interaction, bringing together people from all walks of life. These organizations have allowed people to be willing participants in something larger than their own individual lives, and yet something still sized on a personal scale.

Physical immortality serves a similar function, bringing people together for weekly meetings of varying sizes, longer monthly events, social events, and annual conferences. For me, these gatherings provide a sense of shared community that I find nowhere else in my life.

There is a difference, though, in the quality of my togetherness with others who believe in physical immortality. The community created by traditional religions often seems to be almost an afterthought, an accidental byproduct of bringing people together to worship God. With people believing in physical immortality, though, our sense of togetherness is no accident, but one of our primary goals. We come together, not to worship god, but to worship each other.

Advantages of Physical Immortality

Traditional religions place ultimate responsibility for things in the hands of God. If you believe in a supreme being who is omnipotent, omniscient and omnipresent, then when something goes wrong, you can pretty well bet that it's His fault. This dilutes our responsibility as humans. This belief in God gives us the ultimate excuse, when we do something disliked by another person, of saying that it was "God's will," and that we were only acting as His instrument.

Our responsibility is further reduced by the notion that our time here on earth is only a prelude to a spiritual afterlife. This fosters the belief that whatever we do here on earth is of little consequence, since the real action is in the hereafter.

Traditional religions' view of life here on earth seems to be similar to Charles Barkley's view of the regular season in the National Basketball Association: he calls it the "pre-season." He's learned the hard way that the only goal of regular season play is to make sure you make it to the playoffs. In the same way, many religious followers seem to think that their actions here on earth make little difference, so long as they are sufficient in the eyes of the Lord to grant them admission to heaven.

Physical immortality, in contrast, places all responsibility squarely with us, by counteracting both traditional beliefs. If there is no supreme being outside of ourselves, then we must be responsible, individually and jointly, for what goes on here. And if there is no afterlife, but only more life, then there can be nothing more important than our actions now.

It is this heightened sense of human responsibility that allows us to make the difference here on earth, with ourselves and with each other. It is the willingness to take on this responsibility that gives us the ability to create heaven here on earth.

The Un-Religion

We have seen that physical immortality is like traditional religions in some ways, but radically different from these religions in other ways. At some point, of course, each of us must decide which of these views of reality is true for us.

What's true for me is what works the best. And the belief system that works best in my life is physical immortality. These beliefs make the most difference in the quality of my life today, by giving me the empowerment, the sense of purpose, the faith, the spiritual sense, the values, the responsibility and the people that make a real difference in my life.

For me, immortality has kept all the promises that other religions made but could not keep.

Chapter 30

God

MOST OF US ARE COMFORTABLE with some image of God. These images may differ somewhat, from one person to another, one religion to the next, and one time period to a later one. Yet this image of a singular deity is remarkably pervasive throughout human culture.

This notion of a God has served many functions within the human psyche. We have pictured God as our creator, as the ongoing architect of a divine plan, as a lawgiver, and as our judge.

I believe that many of these ideas we have had about God are unnecessary. All of these images of God have, in different ways, placed arbitrary limits on our vision of our own human potential. By projecting our own traits and abilities onto the image of an external deity, we have deprived ourselves of our own power and dignity.

I have come to realize, though, that God also fulfills a deeper human need.

Unity

As human beings, we are all aware of our independence. We are all capable of living our separate lives. We can each be a law unto ourselves. We can go through life concerned only about our own needs and desires. We can all be self-centered, focused only on our individual lives.

Yet there is something more. We are all aware of being incomplete by ourselves. We all have a sense of being part of a greater whole. We have feelings of harmony in which we are only single notes of a chord, individual instruments within an orchestra, isolated melodies that together make a symphony.

We each have a deep knowing of a greater whole. Just as every cell contains the genetic plan for the entire organism, each one of us has this sense of something bigger, of which we are only a part.

We are like Lego blocks, in a set with no two pieces alike. We can each be separate and disconnected. Yet we sense a potential for something more. Two pieces can be joined together. The combination is interesting, but still leaves us with a feeling of unfulfilled potential. Also like these toy blocks, though, there is no single right way to put us together: only a vast range of exciting possibilities.

I believe we all have these feelings of a grand unity. Yet they can be difficult to articulate, and can seem at odds with the conflicting necessities of everyday life. And these fragile feelings of a deeper connection can easily be chased away by an unkind word, a harsh encounter, or an uncaring response. When surveying the seeming chaos of human affairs, it is often difficult to see a unifying wholeness.

It is easier, though, when we picture this wholeness flowing from a single, pure source. Our images of God, then, have been a way of focusing and intensifying our feelings of oneness. God has served as a symbol that represents these feelings of wholeness, and reminds us of them. If we give this wholeness a name, and project upon it our deepest sense of an overarching unity, then it is easier to feel the larger whole of which we are only parts.

In this sense, then, God is like a mantra, or candle, that serves as an object for our meditation. The value is not in the object itself, but only in its ability to focus our thoughts and feelings.

Organized Religion

There is another useful way to extend our Lego block analogy. As you will remember, individual humans are like the blocks, with the potential to be connected in a greater whole. Organized religions, then, are like the sheets of instructions that tell you how to put the blocks together in a particular way. The value of such specific directions, as any Lego engineer will tell you, is in the reliability of the plan. Someone else has already tried and tested the design, and if you follow it religiously, then you are sure to achieve an impressive result.

The problem, of course, is in the rigidity of such an approach. If you take the instructions that come with the set as your bible, then you will only be able to build a single design. If you hold that single image pictured on the front of the box as sacred, then you will never advance beyond that one model.

Yet other designs are possible. If you have two or more kits, then you can build even grander designs by combining pieces from the different sets. Even one large kit can be used to make a virtually unlimited number of possible configurations.

Manifesting God

God has been a sort of middleman for human togetherness. By having many people focus on a common image of God, human beings have grown closer to one another. By following commandments supposedly handed down by God, people have been able to live together in constructive human society. By cherishing the noble ideals embodied in an image of God, we have nourished and supported each other and made it a joy to be human.

God and religion have had grand functions. They have served their purposes. Yet they have also created confusion. We have worshipped the picture on the front of the box, instead of our own feelings of wholeness. We have insisted that there was only one right way to bring people together, when in fact there are many possibilities.

What would it be like to eliminate the middleman? To me, it is the greatest pleasure to feel this connection directly with other people. It is the greatest joy to feel this sense of wholeness arise directly from myself and those around me. It is wondrous delight to know that I am a vital part of a larger human community.

Chapter 31

The New Age

WHILE TRADITIONAL RELIGIOUS BELIEFS have been on the decline lately, something called the New Age movement has been growing in popularity over the last few years. You may be wondering whether physical immortality is part of this movement, or something altogether different.

It is hard to find any precise definition of the New Age belief system. There is no official body to resolve contradictions, and make official decrees. In fact, one of the defining elements of the New Age movement seems to be that it is a grab-bag of alternative beliefs, an accumulation of techniques, rather than a cohesive whole.

I've made an attempt, though, to summarize the defining beliefs of the New Age movement, as I see them. They are listed below. After the statement of each belief, I will discuss similarities and differences with beliefs founded on human physical immortality.

As with many types of beliefs, there are often differences between the best forms of these ideas and common misconceptions. I'll try to acknowledge both variations in my discussion of New Age principles.

1. Humanity is moving towards some sort of "New Age," some new phase of human life on this planet.

I agree about the possibility of a new and more enlightened era dawning for humanity.

The best New Age authors emphasize that it is up to each of us to make this new era come to pass. This belief is often misinterpreted, however, to mean that this benevolent unfolding is predestined by some higher power. People mistakenly assume that it will inevitably happen, whether or not we as individual humans do anything to advance it.

I do believe that humanity has reached a point at which it has started to uncover new possibilities for human existence. This movement towards a higher consciousness, though, is no more than the collective movement of enlightened human beings. There is no outside force coordinating the unfolding of this new age, or determining its nature. It is up to each of us to make it happen, and to determine what it will look like.

2. There is a spiritual dimension of our existence that has been overlooked and underdeveloped.

Again I see basic agreement. Modern humans have become too focused on things we can see and measure with precision, and we need to develop qualities of ourselves that are unseen. Spirit is that which produces life, and we need to devote ourselves more to pursuits that increase our liveliness.

At issue, though, is the nature of this spiritual dimension. Some New Age believers see spirit as a pure substance that is separate from, and superior to, our gross physical existence. They believe that spirit infuses the flesh, but that pure spirit, and spiritual beings, can exist on their own. This naturally leads to an unnecessary separation between spirit and flesh, between the sacred and the profane, between god and man.

It is true that there is a mystery about the attributes of humanity that are called "spiritual." This mystery naturally arises because these spiritual attributes are subtle and unseen. We can see how tall someone is, and the color of their hair. It is harder to determine whether they are gentle or mean, boisterous or quiet, thoughtful or impulsive.

I think that these hidden attributes have been made too mysterious, though. Although this "spiritual" dimension of our existence is not yet thoroughly explained by science, there is no reason to think that it comes from any source outside of our very material selves. We are spirit as well as flesh, but there is no spirit apart from flesh.

Many people, especially those who have been following spiritual pursuits for some time, see their physical forms as imperfect and limited. It almost seems that the more they devote themselves to spiritual concerns, the more imperfect their ordinary physical lives become.

These "spiritual" types remind me of those who habitually play high-stakes lotteries. They can become so focused on what they could do with a million dollars, that their current financial situations seem impossibly limited by comparison.

If you devote yourself to fantasy, then reality will always pale by comparison.

I don't really believe in the possibility of a purely spiritual existence. Some people picture themselves becoming bodies of pure energy. To me, this sounds like driving a car that is pure gasoline. Energy is great, but I'm not sure how far it would take me if I didn't have a little matter to go with it.

Even if I consider the possibility of a purely spiritual existence, though, I'm not really attracted to the idea. I like being flesh and blood. I like substance. I like the feel of wind upon my face. I like the touch of another human being, the sensation of skin upon skin. I can't imagine living without it. What's more, I can't imagine *wanting* to live without it.

For me, I find my physical existence to be unlimited. I find that my life contains more possibilities than I could ever have imagined.

The secret, I have found, lies in other people. By myself, no matter how wonderful I am, I will eventually find my boundaries, my limitations. But when I join with others, then I find myself no longer bound by my personal limitations. With other people, I find that I can do and become anything that I really want.

3. There is some new form of energy at work in the universe, other than those already recognized by mainstream science.

There is always this possibility. Efforts to define the nature of this energy, or confirm its existence, have been remarkably inconsistent, however.

One crucial distinction that needs to be made here is between the laws of physics and the "laws" describing the actions and interactions of living organisms.

New Age believers are fond of talking about the "universe." They often speak of universal laws. They speak of the universe as a conscious entity, and ascribe intelligence to this thing. They speak of the universe "giving to them."

It is well to remember that the actual universe consists largely of empty space, interrupted occasionally by unspeakably hot stars, surrounded at safe distances by huge orbiting rocks. In general, not a very friendly place for human beings. The laws describing the behavior of these objects are the laws of physics, which are getting rather well known, and do not seem to include such mysterious energies as are popular with New Age believers.

These attributes that New Agers project on the universe, however, begin to make a lot more sense when we see them as qualities of living organisms, especially primates, and most particularly human beings. And whereas the laws of physics are rather stable and well-known to scientists, we are only beginning to scratch the surface of all the various ways in which living organisms can behave. So let's look at human capacities for traces of some "mysterious energy."

It is true that all of us have thoughts, feelings and impulses whose origins are often mysterious to us. We may find ourselves at the right place at the right time, without the slightest clue as to how we came to be there. We may make a decision without really knowing why, and later discover some wonderful benefit that we were unconscious of at the time, or some terrible tragedy that would have befallen us if we had made another choice.

Are events like these the products of pure chance? Are they rather the results of subconscious perceptions and thoughts going on underneath the surfaces of our minds? Or are they evidence of some unseen energy at work, some hidden synchronicity?

At times, there is no doubt that such coincidences really are the result of dumb luck. There is a certain amount of chance at work in the universe, and all sorts of superstitious beliefs have been devised over the centuries based on such happenstance. This is not to say, however, that all such occurrences are products of pure chance.

There is also no doubt that our minds sometimes work in ways we do not understand. Human reasoning has produced such wonderful results that we are at times a bit too enthralled with it. When we have thoughts or feelings that are not the results of conscious reasoning, we sometimes grow suspicious of them. Yet these impulses often prove correct, even though it may not be until later, if ever, that we understand how these ideas came to us.

There is nothing magical or implausible about such beliefs. It is not irrational to trust our intuition, even though these thoughts may not have come to us through the process of conscious reasoning. This would be like refusing to watch television, because we do not understand the technical details of how it works.

So some of these "synchronous" events can be assumed to be products of chance, and others the results of human intuition. Is there also a third category, some events that can only be explained by some reference to an unknown force?

Perhaps. It is a little dangerous, though, to assume the existence of such a force. For one thing, this energy is commonly viewed as having its source outside of human beings. Such separation typically leads to abdication of human responsibility, and projection of our own human qualities upon the universe.

It seems safer, to me, to ascribe such synchronicity to our own very human qualities. I don't really believe in mysterious forces outside of ourselves – until, at least, they can be proven. I do believe, though, in mysterious forces at work within us: "mysterious," that is, in the sense that we are not fully aware of how these forces operate.

We are more powerful than we know, or than we are willing to admit. Much of the excitement of living forever lies in exploring the untapped potential that is within each one of us, and within the infinite connections between us.

4. We need to let go of dysfunctional patterns in our lives that we have unconsciously inherited from past lives and childhood experiences.

Agreed. Although there is some distinction to be made about how we are to get beyond these old patterns.

One strategy is to constantly work on ourselves, analyzing our patterns so that we can free ourselves from them. This is the onion approach, always peeling off one layer only to find another waiting below.

The immortal strategy is to transcend these patterns by becoming conscious of a creative aliveness that is outside of these patterns. We can then allow ourselves to be energized by this aliveness.

5. It is time for human beings to form relationships with each other based on cooperation and co-creation, rather than on power struggles and competition.

Yes! Absolutely! Couldn't agree more.

Again, though, there is a subtle trap here. It is a mistake to passively "go with the flow," rather than fully expressing one's individuality. Our culture has tended to portray individuality and togetherness as incompatible opposites. From this mistaken point of view, one can be a "rugged individual," or one can conform to others' expectations in order to fit in to a larger society.

There is a better way, though. If we recognize each person as different and valid, yet limited, then we can create a togetherness made up of the best of each of us, while still preserving our individuality. We should not all have to agree on everything – or even pretend we do – in order to cooperate and work together. When we acknowledge the strengths and weaknesses that all of us have, we should be able to contribute in areas where we are strong, and go along with others in areas where they are stronger.

The best example I can offer is my six-year stint at editing a magazine about physical immortality. In the early issues, I did everything myself: editing, layout and cover design. I enjoyed all of these activities, and was pleased with the results. As the magazine grew, I relied more and more on the contributions of others. As we continued to work together, we discovered what worked and what didn't. What never worked, for me, was abdication of responsibility. I couldn't simply compromise my own strong beliefs, or go along with someone else just to be a nice guy. For example, if someone submitted an article that I didn't feel would work, I had to tell them so.

At the same time, though, I found that it sometimes worked

to trust others in areas where they were strong. My specialty was to select and shape the words that went into the magazine. Doug Morris, a good friend from England, became responsible for the layout, for the overall look of the publication. There were sometimes decisions in these areas where we disagreed. It wasn't that I didn't have feelings in these areas – I always had an opinion! In cases, though, where my feelings were not particularly strong, and weren't based on any absolute principles, I found that it worked to yield to Doug on these sorts of issues. When I say that it worked, I don't just mean that it made Doug happy – I mean that it resulted in a better magazine. I saw that other people liked the magazine more. I even noticed that the magazine looked better to me! I discovered that we worked better as a team when I recognized my own limitations, and his strengths.

Yet there were other times when I had strong feelings about design issues, sometimes in areas where Doug did not. And, at times, I made these decisions, even when Doug mildly disagreed. So there were no hard and fast rules, no absolute divisions of responsibility. Instead, there was this constant teamwork, ongoing cooperation, and continuing learning, even when we disagreed.

This sort of cooperation and co-creation isn't always easy, and is never wishy-washy, but it is definitely a quantum leap over old modes of competition.

6. We are part of something greater than ourselves. We are conscious of our connection to all things.

I agree that our true nature is to be connected, to be part of a greater whole, and not to be isolated and separate.

At the same time, though, it is a trap to think that this something greater will go on unaffected without us.

There are two sorts of models here, and it is crucial that we get them straight. One sort of feeling is to be part of something made from an accumulation of identical units. An example would be to feel like a drop of water in the ocean of life. The ocean is made of a vast number of such drops, but all the drops are the same. If one drop is lost, then the ocean will still exist essentially unchanged, except for being imperceptibly and infinitesimally smaller.

The other sort of model is an organic one. This is the feeling of being an organ in a living body. Every organ is different. Some are smaller than others. Yet remove any one, and the functioning of the body as a whole is damaged, if not stopped altogether. In this model, there is a synergistic effect. The whole is greater than the sum of the parts.

If we see ourselves as a drop of water, then we may feel part of something greater, but we will be mistaken about the importance of our role in that greater whole. It is essential that we see ourselves as essential organs, that make a vital difference in the functioning of the whole.

Part X

What We See in the Mirror

32. A New Self-Image

When we acknowledge the human potential for physical immortality, it causes a profound change in the way we view ourselves, as individuals and collectively as human beings. This chapter builds on everything that has come before it, and summarizes this new way of looking at ourselves.

Chapter 32

A New Self-Image

OUR COLLECTIVE HUMAN SELF-IMAGE has radically changed at times in the past. We once thought that the sun and stars revolved around us. Our discovery that the earth is not the center of the universe, then, was one cause for a sobering reappraisal of our place in the cosmos. More recently, Darwin's assertion that we are descended from apes has again altered our view of what it means to be human.

Acknowledgment of our potential for immortality has the power to again transform our view of humanity. Following are the major elements of this new self-appraisal.

1. **Humanity is the major creative force at work in the universe today.**

We are not the products of an omniscient god, or even an intelligent universe. We are the products of evolution. And while evolution has proven itself to be an immensely creative process, it is also tremendously slow, using trial and error in place of intelligent anticipation or conscious desire.

Human beings, on the other hand, do possess conscious desire and are capable of intelligent anticipation, with our growing knowledge of causes and their effects. For better or worse, we are increasingly becoming the architects of planet earth. It is not that we are responsible for everything that is here. For example, we didn't create the mountains and oceans, and all the many forms of life on the planet, let alone the rest of the universe. But we are changing things faster than any other force at work today.

Along with this realization of our creative role on a global scale, comes the acceptance of our parts as creators at a more personal level. There are many things in our lives that we want and value – not just material things, but qualities of life, like peace and happiness. For ease of discussion, let me refer to the sum of these things we desire as our prosperity. As human beings, though, we are not passive recipients of what prosperity we possess – we are the creators of it. Most, if not all, of the things we desire for ourselves are things that we ourselves can create – if not individually, then as part of a larger human collective.

I am speaking, not at a metaphysical level, but at a very practical and physical level. Do you want love? This is something created by humans. Do you want wood, to build a house? This is something grown and harvested by humans. Do you want a peaceful existence? Barring natural disasters, the effects of which can be mitigated by humans, peace is something created by humans.

2. Every person alive today has the potential for immortality.

This is true for every person still breathing, no matter how old they are, no matter where they come from, no matter what their skin color, no matter what their current medical condition may be. There is no death sentence placed on any of us. We are immortal until proven otherwise.

3. We are not perfect, and neither are we striving to attain perfection.

We can only determine the perfection of something by comparing it to a known standard. In order for something to be perfect, we have to know what class of things it belongs to, and what the function of that class is.

But there is no outside authority capable of defining a standard by which to measure human beings. And since part of the value of each of us lies in our uniqueness, there is no universal standard possible.

4. Every human being is unique and infinitely valuable.

We are essentially different from every other species of life on earth. We have reached a point in our development at which our greatest strength comes, not from having masses of people all performing the same function, but from having as many different types of people as possible.

Humanity is not a bee hive. We are not divided into queen bees and workers, with every worker performing the same function. Even in areas where we seem to benefit from being alike, this is usually an illusion created by looking at ourselves from too great a distance, or in too abstract a sense.

Let me give you one example. I worked for a large corporation for many years. We had several thousand people working at our location. From the point of view of upper management, or of the human resources department, each person fit into a certain job description. From this perspective, all people working at the same job performed the same function, and required the same knowledge, skills and aptitudes to be successful.

In actual practice, though, everyone I ever knew there had a slightly different job, performed unique functions, and possessed distinct qualifications. We were all different. And it was our differences that made us work effectively as a company. If I was weak in one area, then someone else would be strong. Individually we were very fallible. As a whole, though, we were much more than the sum of our parts, and were immensely powerful and effective.

5. We all deserve to live forever.

Every person on the planet deserves to live. Every one of us is worthy. No one is disposable. There is no age at which our status changes. There is no condition that can diminish our worth. There is no sin we can commit that can cause our value to be revoked.

The US Declaration of Independence asserts that all people have inalienable rights to "life, liberty and the pursuit of happiness." We often take this right to life for granted, as if it didn't mean much. But an inalienable right to life means that we deserve to live as much when we have been here for 200 years, as when we are two or 20.

6. We are constantly changing and evolving.

As a whole, humanity is growing and changing at an unprecedented rate. Even though our physical equipment is still evolving relatively slowly, the cultural software that makes us what we are is changing at an astonishing pace.

Individually, each of us is also changing and evolving. We are learning new things, changing our opinions, developing new tastes, and contributing to society in new ways.

7. We determine our own purpose.

Since there is no God, there is no divine plan. Since there is no universal intelligence that created us, there is no manifest destiny for us to fulfill.

This is not to say that our lives are without purpose. It is, instead, to say that it is up to us to determine our own purpose. This is true individually and collectively. In other words, it is up to each of us to determine the purpose of humanity, and to declare our own role within this larger movement.

The result of this kind of thinking is the most radical form of humanism.

My dictionary defines humanism as, first: "A system of thought that centers on human beings and their values, capacities, and worth." Second, it defines humanism as: "Concern with the interests, needs, and welfare of human beings."

Is our purpose in life to have the best collection of baseball cards in the world? To create a work of art that moves people in profound ways? To make one other person feel loved? To create heaven on earth? No one can say that any one purpose is more valid than another. It is up to each of us to define the purpose of our lives, individually and with each other.

8. We are the higher power we have been looking for.

Throughout human history, we have imagined the existence of some higher power. We have called it God, or the Universe. We have seen this force as immensely powerful. We have seen ourselves as connected to this higher power, or as part of it. We have seen its workings as mysterious, and have seen ourselves as unable to comprehend this higher power in its entirety.

In a very practical sense, what comes closest to meeting

these characteristics is ourselves: humanity as a whole. We are, collectively, the major creative force at work in the universe. As people working together, we are immensely powerful: capable of altering the face of the earth, and of sending people to the moon. As individuals, we are connected to, and part of, the whole of humanity.

And, in the largest sense, the workings of humanity are mysterious, and incapable of being fully understood by any one individual. Because we are all different and unique, and because there are so many of us, there is no one individual who can fully comprehend the workings of humanity as a whole. It is not possible to understand the distinct contributions of each member of the human race.

Together, we comprise all the attributes we have for so long projected on a distant higher power. For each of us, it is true that there is a power "higher" than our individual selves: it is the power of two, three or more of us when we come together.

9. We are part of the universe, and part of life on earth.

All this talk about humanity should not leave the impression that we are alone or self-sufficient. We are part of the universe, composed of the same sub-atomic particles as stars and planets. We are residents of planet earth, and of the solar system in which this planet orbits. And we are connected to all life on earth, sharing many characteristics with all other species of life. And our lives are made possible only by a complex interdependence between all these things.

10. We are capable of creating heaven on earth.

A friend of mine once said that, "Heaven is right here with one another, and hell is six feet under."

Once we dispense with religious mythology, and acknowledge that we have the potential to stay alive forever, then the possibility of an earthbound Eden takes on new meaning.

It is up to us to define what we mean by "heaven." But, however we define it, it is within our grasp to create it here on earth with one another.

Part XI

Applied Immortality

This section gives some practical examples of how I've applied the principles of living forever to other areas of my life.

Chapter 33. Immortal Parenting

How does living forever affect the process of having and raising a child? It's had a lot of positive impact, in my case.

Chapter 34. Rebirthing

The possibility of physical immortality has also changed the way I think about giving and receiving bodywork.

Chapter 33

Immortal Parenting

LIVING FOREVER IS A DECISION that has affected all aspects of my life. For many people, the idea of physical immortality seems to have little to do with the realities of everyday living. Yet this act of embracing my own endlessness has made many concrete differences in my life, including my attitudes and actions as a parent.

Conception

Pauline and I had been together for several years before we decided we wanted to have a child. As it turned out, making this decision, and subsequently abandoning our attempts at birth control, were not enough to make our intention a reality. We tried to conceive for a couple of years, while living in Los Angeles, without any success.

Then, on February 1, 1986, we moved to Mesa, Arizona as the result of a job relocation. There we met three extraordinary people: Charles Paul Brown, Bernadeane Brown, and James Russell Strole. They were founders of an organization called People Forever, and held regular weekly meetings on the subject of physical immortality. Pauline became pregnant soon after, and our son Stephen, was born on February 1, 1987. Mere coincidence? I don't think so. Pauline, even more than I, was hungry for these people. At some level she was looking for them. Something in her was not ready to have a baby without knowing that she had these people in her life: people who would support us and our child in unlimited aliveness. The first effect that physical immortality had on me as a parent, then, was that it enabled me to become one.

The Family Structure

A lasting desire for physical immortality is not possible without a deep feeling that people are more important than anything else. When death is seen as inevitable, though, people are seen as subordinate to the institutions that outlast them. The family is the most enduring of these institutions. Within the system of death, the family becomes more important than its individual members. In this context, relatives are often valued primarily for the roles they play within the family structure.

There has been much discussion in recent years about freeing women from their traditional roles as mothers and housewives. There has also been some attention paid to the restrictions of the traditional male role model. Children have been included in these discussions in terms of their sexuality, and the effect that these male/female role models have on their developing personalities.

What has *not* been discussed is the role of children within the family – *as* children. The tragic results have been modern families in which the parents have been liberated from their traditional roles, but the children are still enslaved.

Multiplication

The traditional Biblical injunction is to "Be fruitful, and multiply...."[45] In a world of death, one of the primary functions of children is propagation of the species. Children are the pawns in an evolutionary struggle for survival of the fittest. It is only logical, in this context, to have as many as possible.

Because I don't see myself as dying, I see no need to produce children in order to ensure the survival of my species. My decision to have a child was based on my desire to have a unique new individual in my life. Stephen has satisfied this desire for me. I have no interest in having more children. I don't feel the need to have a "big family." I don't feel the need to have a family of any size – the need I feel is for particular individuals: Pauline and Stephen.

Similarly, I am not worried about losing Stephen, so I don't feel moved to have more children, in case something "should happen" to him. We are not accidents on our way to happen. Stephen is here with me forever.

Reproduction

Another function of children has been to carry on the family name – and the family genetic material. For parents who expect to die, children are a means of achieving some sort of immortality. The mother and father may perish, but some part of them will live on in their children, and in their children's children.

In this situation, the role of the child is to be as similar as possible to the parents. Parents often expect their children to be like them. Every emerging feature, or personality trait, is carefully examined in hopes that it will mirror a similar characteristic of one of the child's parents. Boys are expected to be like their fathers, and girls like their mothers. Deviations from the parental characteristics are discouraged, and suppressed, if possible.

As a man who was born on his father's birthday, and named after him as a result, I suppose I have been particularly sensitive to this issue. In any case, I have not had any desire to see Stephen become a little Herb. I can certainly see some of my characteristics, and some of Pauline's, in our son. I am excited, though, and not disappointed, when I also note differences – ways in which Stephen is uniquely himself.

Since I'm not going anywhere, I don't need another me. I see every person, including my son, as infinitely valuable precisely because he is like no other. I love Stephen for the person he is, and for the person he is becoming.

No Favorite Age

I frequently hear people confess that they love children at a certain age. Mothers often prefer infants, while fathers sometimes favor children who are older, and therefore easier to interact with as adults.

This sort of confession often comes from a parent whose children have all passed their favorite age group. Sometimes these parents seem to be lost in wistful memories of their children as infants. Others seem to be critical of their own children at their current, dissatisfying, ages, or to have lost touch with them, as if they were no longer of interest. Others (surprise!) shortly announce that they have another little one on the way, and look forward expectantly to being able to relive their earlier experiences with their other children. (These same parents, of course, are usually dismayed and disappointed when their lovely babies grow up into alienated teenagers.)

I have never felt this kind of age preference. I've enjoyed Stephen at all of his ages. He is now ten, and I feel no sentimental fondness for him as a baby. I think he gets more wonderful all the time. Most of all, though, my appreciation for him continues to grow, the more I get to know him. I fully expect to enjoy him even more when he is fourteen, and more again when he is twenty.

Our Relationship

From the beginning, I have related to Stephen as one individual to another, and not as a parent to a child. Stephen, for me, is – and always has been – a person. I don't expect him to act a certain way, because this is the way children are supposed to act, or because this is the way our family acts.

I believe that most of the problems that parents have with children are caused by the parents' attempts to find one "right" way to "deal with" children. Every child is different. There is no one "right" way to treat all children, just as there is no one "right" way to treat all adults, or all men, or all women. And children are not problems that we as parents need to "deal with" – they are people we want to enjoy.

It is not always easy to treat people as individuals. It is a demanding and challenging activity. In the long run, though, it is a lot more fun to have a bunch of interesting individuals in your life, than to have a lot of people imperfectly acting out various roles that you have scripted for them. In the case of my son Stephen, this attitude towards him has resulted in a tremendous and ever growing enjoyment of him.

Rules

People often have rigid rules for children. Some of these rules are important, but others are based on false images of the way children are supposed to act.

I remember a weekend when Pauline's parents were out to visit. We were driving in the car, and Stephen was in the back seat with his grandparents. Stephen was talking about a friend who had gotten in trouble for using "bad" words. Pauline's father, Clendon, who is a terrible tease, saw his opportunity. Feigning the utmost innocence, he said, "Oh, yeah, what kind of words?" Stephen, sidestepping this invitation to repeat the profanities, politely said that the words were "dirty."

This response opened up a new line of attack. Clendon made the assumption that Stephen had not used the words in question because he, too, would get in trouble for saying them. With Pauline and myself only a few feet away, Clendon now felt safe in repeating his question several times, pressing Stephen for more details, and playfully frustrating him in the process.

Stephen tolerated the questions a couple more times and then – since Clendon seemed to really want to know – calmly uttered a couple of words that made Clendon blush, as he sank down into his seat. Pauline and I just smiled.

We have realized for some time that it is impossible to keep Stephen from hearing these sorts of words. Forbidding him to repeat them would be silly, for a number of reasons. First, the words by themselves cause no harm. Second, forbidding their use implies that they have some sort of magical power, making them an irresistible temptation. Third, telling him to never use these words would also make them more attractive as a means of asserting his independence. Finally, we have no way of preventing him from using them when he is among friends, so the rule would be impossible to enforce.

Our alternative has been to simply explain to Stephen that some people don't like to hear these words, especially from children. He has understood this easily, and has never offended anyone by using them – except when directly asked to, as in the case with his grandfather.

Rules are important at times, but people are fundamentally more important than rules. This attitude has made it fairly easy for us to avoid imposing double standards, and rules that have no meaning.

In Summary

I don't mean to give you the impression that I believe myself to be a perfect parent, or that I think Stephen a perfect child. Being a parent – and being a human being – is a process of growth and discovery. I've said and done things that I've later regretted (and probably a few that I may yet wish I could undo).

I do believe, though, that physical immortality has given me a distinct advantage in being a parent. It's taken my son and me out of the family structure, and out of the struggle for survival, and allowed us both to appreciate each other as people. And since people are the most important things in the world, for both of us, this immortal attitude tends to put everything else in the proper perspective.

Chapter 34

Rebirthing

REBIRTHING IS A BREATHING TECHNIQUE that enhances one's feelings of aliveness, helps to integrate all parts of ourselves, and can reawaken early memories, back to and including recollections of one's birth. The process was discovered by Leonard Orr, and popularized by others such as Sondra Ray and Colin Sisson. All three of these individuals have also spoken about the possibility of physical immortality, and so the practice of rebirthing has become associated with the promise of living forever. Rebirthing is often performed with a guide or facilitator, known as a rebirther. My wife Pauline and I were both trained as rebirthers. Many of the following comments could also be applied to other forms of counseling and bodywork.

When Pauline and I first experienced rebirthing, we were already aware of the possibility of physical immortality. As our ideas and experience grew, though, we gradually changed our perception of the importance of the presence of another living human being versus the value of technique.

What do I mean by physical immortality? I mean the feeling that we are meant to be here, forever, in our physical bodies. I mean putting an end to all separation between people, including the separation of death. I mean accepting the physical body and the soul as two different terms for the same reality, and ending the belief that the body is a disposable container for the immortal soul. I mean believing in physical immortality as our own personal destiny, and not just some abstract potentiality for mankind. I mean accepting each other, just as we are, as being totally enough for each other, as being the nourishment we need to keep each other throughout eternity. This is physical immortality as I have come to know it.

How does all this affect the rebirthing process? First, it makes the people as important as the process. Without immortality, the rebirther is often viewed as a mere guide to the process of rebirthing. Immortality restores the rebirther-rebirthee relationship to primacy, and makes the process a technique for magnifying, amplifying, and focusing the intimacy of that relationship. Physical immortality puts the breathing process in the proper perspective, and empowers the rebirther and rebirthee to really make the difference with each other.

Seen in this light, rebirthing is a way of heightening the intimacy between the people involved. This intimacy is vitally important to rebirthing. It is this deep cellular contact that creates an atmosphere of safety and trust, in which the rebirthee feels free to totally let down all barriers and defenses.

Intimacy cannot be total until all threats of separation are removed. To fully heal the birth trauma, the rebirthee must realize that the ultimate closeness felt before birth, between the child and its mother, is not some garden of Eden from which we are ejected. Rather, it is an earnest of our inheritance, it is the condition in which life is meant to be lived.

The promise of that initial intimacy must be fulfilled by the relationship between the rebirther and the rebirthee. To make this fulfillment possible, the threat of death, the ultimate separation, must be removed. As long as the possibility of the death of one of the participants remains, then the rebirthee will always hold some part of himself back. He will refrain from total surrender, and will not be able to heal his first loss. Immortals are free to give themselves away totally, because they know their investment can never be lost.

It is important to note that the intimacy we are speaking of is not a one-way street. The rebirther must be willing to let down all barriers, to go all the way, to risk as much, or more, than the rebirthee. This requires a total commitment to physical immortality on the part of both participants.

A belief in mortal spirituality, in a god outside of us that is our source, only furthers a sense of separation. If you feel that your connection with god is the primary relationship in your life, that god is your starting and ending point, then you will reserve your total intimacy for god. If, on the other hand, you believe as an immortal that your fellow man is the ultimate manifestation of god, then you will invest yourself totally in your relationships here on earth.

A belief in death further contributes to separation. To achieve total intimacy, you must be willing to go all the way with each other, to fully be all that you are in each other's presence. If you believe in your own mortality, however, then you believe that your physical body is transient, and your soul is your ultimate reality. You probably believe that you are here to learn some spiritual lesson, and once that is complete, you will be free to shed your body and return to your original and ultimate condition.

In other words, for a mortal, going all the way literally means dying! What a block to realizing your full potential! In contrast, with an immortal consciousness, going all the way always means plunging deeper and deeper into life, and into each other.

Rebirthing is often seen as a way of releasing negativity. Immortality expands this role. To be willing to live forever, one must always have new horizons to look forward to. With this in mind, rebirthing can be seen as a way of facilitating our continual expansion, our always plunging further into our unlimited depths.

Immortality is a physical experience that can only be realized through contact with other immortals, with those able to draw out the immortal response in the cells of your own body. The acceptance of physical immortality has transformed my experience of the process of rebirthing.

Part XII

Where To Go From Here ...

In the last part of this book, I share with you some possibilities for further development of your immortality. You'll find some suggestions for what to do next, now that you have all eternity to look forward to!

Chapter 35. Immortality and You

There are various attitudes you can take towards the possibility of physical immortality, and some are more useful than others.

Chapter 36. Seven Ways to Change the World

Can we really change the world? Here are seven solid ideas for doing so that I haven't had time to work on yet. Feel free to take one of these and run with it. Or come up with your own. Just so long as you don't "go with the flow." (Isn't that a waterfall I hear up ahead?)

Chapter 37. Next Steps

Hopefully, by now, I've convinced you there's a better way to live. How do you start out in this new life? I offer a few suggestions.

Chapter 35

Immortality and You

Making It Personal

IF YOU HAVE THE SLIGHTEST INTEREST IN PHYSICAL IMMORTALITY, then you need to determine the nature of your relationship with it. Like all relationships, yours with immortality will change and evolve over time. It is worthwhile, though, to examine the nature of this association consciously and intentionally. Your primary attitude towards immortality can take many different forms. Let's look at many of the common ones and the differing implications of each.

1. I'll wait and see what happens.

Physical immortality is all about taking personal responsibility, so waiting for someone or something else to make it happen is not likely to produce any positive results in your own life. I've actually heard people say, "If you're still around one hundred years from now, then come look me up and we'll talk about immortality then." The only problem, of course, is that

I'll probably have to look you up in the graveyard, and it's likely to be a one-sided conversation!

The fallacy with this attitude is the notion that we can afford to wait. We can't, of course. Waiting to see about immortality is like sitting in a boat, drifting towards a waterfall, and waiting to see if you really need to row. By the time you're sure you need to, it'll be too late for your actions to have much effect.

2. Immortality sounds like a good idea, and is something that will probably come to pass in the future.

This attitude can take a few different forms. You may believe that God will bring about physical immortality when He is good and ready. Or you may think that some other impersonal force, like evolution or nature, will cause immortality to happen someday. Or you may see immortality as something that will eventually be realized by medical science.

There are several questions worth asking here. If immortality is to come about someday, then why not now? What is God, or evolution, or humanity waiting for?

And if some force bigger than you is going to make immortality happen, then what does this force need *you* for? Why do you need to be immortal, if you are not yourself this bigger force?

And, finally, if you care about living forever, then why leave it up to others to bring it about? Why not fully commit yourself to making it happen?

3. Immortality sounds like an interesting option, and I like to keep all my options open. I'll decide later.

This approach reminds me of the smoker who says he can quit anytime he wants to – he just doesn't want to yet. We all know that there are situations in which deciding not to make a decision is itself a decision. This is one of those cases.

People often have the illusion that death is a single event. The truth is that it is a slow, gradual process. Whether people die from sudden accidents, or long lingering illnesses, the final termination of life is the culmination of a process that began long ago.

Every moment that we are alive, we are either taking another step towards eternity, or another step towards the grave. It is up to us to choose a direction, but it is a decision that we make every day, whether we own up to it or not.

4. I'm definitely going to live forever – either physically or spiritually – but there's no urgency about deciding which way I want to go.

It is true that there is a feeling of eternity that can come from a belief in an afterlife, as well as from a commitment to physical immortality.

A belief in an afterlife can also lull us into a false sense of security, though. This is precisely why Karl Marx said that "Religion … is the opium of the masses."[46] It is altogether too easy to look forward to a wonderful hereafter, no matter what is going on in the here and now.

It is more demanding – and more rewarding – to decide to create your own heaven right here on earth. Then you look clearly at what you are creating for yourself, and eliminate any excuses for why your everyday reality looks different from your ultimate goal.

5. Immortality is a wonderful goal, and I will strive to continually improve myself until I one day achieve it.

If immortality is viewed as a state of perfection, then it will become unachievable – the tasty carrot that is always hanging just out of reach. If you are improving yourself in order to achieve immortality, then you will never be quite good enough.

If you are striving to achieve immortality, then you will also set up a polarity between who you are now, and who you want to be, that will keep you locked into your present reality. Like a dieter who is always telling himself that he needs to lose weight, you will be unconsciously reinforcing your current reality. If you want to lose weight, then you need to begin visualizing yourself as already slim, and affirming that you easily maintain your ideal weight. Then your reality will tend to correct itself to match your vision of who you already see yourself to be.

Saying you're going to achieve immortality is like a dolphin saying she's going to the ocean. If you're on dry land, then the ocean may be a destination. For a dolphin, though, the ocean is a condition of its existence, the space in which it exists, and the medium that allows it to go anywhere at all.

6. I don't have to do anything to live forever – I just have to accept myself as already immortal.

I have heard people say that they are immortal – even though they smoke habitually, or are obese, or never bother to exercise. I have no desire to try to convince these people that they are merely mortal – on the contrary, I may believe in their immortality even more than they do. It is dangerous, though, to disconnect our current condition and our everyday actions from our immortality. If we are living in this sort of dream, than we are no better off than having some hazy vision of an afterlife.

Many people have had silly and juvenile images of heaven – pink Cadillacs driving down streets paved with gold, for example. It is easy, though, to have equally immature notions of immortality.

It is pleasant to indulge ourselves in fantasies of wish-fulfillment. We can see ourselves as immortal in the same way that we see ourselves winning the lottery, or drinking too much with no thought of the next morning's hangover, or eating ice cream and cake with no feeling for the long term effects these foods are having on us.

Enjoying ourselves and others are important parts of being immortal. Yet immortality requires more than instant sensory gratification. If we believe that we can do anything we want, whenever we want to do it – now that we have decided that we are immortal – then we are only kidding ourselves.

7. Immortality is something I already am, something that makes me yearn for more, and something I am creating for myself on a daily basis.

This seems to be the healthiest relationship with immortality.

If I am not immortal now, then I never will be. I am as immortal now as I'm ever going to get.

Immortality is not a fixed and final state, however. It is not just a different destination than the grave – it is an altogether different *sort* of destination. Immortality is a hunger for more, a hunger that can only be satisfied by more time, more opportunity to become and to create. Immortality is not what I am trying to become, but it is the freedom and the desire to constantly become more. My eternity is the field in which I always become anew.

It may seem like a paradox to say that physical immortality is both something that gives me the freedom to create, and what I am creating. Yet it has only been our deep duality, our own separation from ourselves, that has made us see cause and effect as two different things. Does the ocean come from the skies, or does the rain come from the sea? Is it plants that are dependent on the carbon dioxide from animals, or beasts that could not live without the oxygen from photosynthesis?

My immortality is a spring constantly renewing itself, a Phoenix ever rising from its own ashes. Creation is the verb, and I am both the subject and the object.

Chapter 36

Seven Ways to Change the World

MANY PEOPLE TODAY HAVE GROWN CYNICAL about our ability to change the world. Self-help is big business, but there often seems to be no help for the world at large. The same person who may be losing weight, working out, and doing affirmations to improve their beliefs may not even find enough time to vote. The world seems so large, and to have so much inertia, that it sometimes seems impossible to change.

Yet this is not the immortal way. Immortal transformation starts with an individual, but it extends outwards from there to include the entire world. You begin by changing yourself, and your private life, but you don't stop until you have transformed the world to fully support an immortal quality of life for every human being on the planet. An immortal life is one without limitations, and one of maximum connection to others, so it is not possible to stake out some small area for yourself, and then be content with that.

Unlike many people, I can think of so many ways to change the world that I can't find enough time to do them all. So I am offering seven suggestions here. I think all these ideas are practical and useful, so at the very least I hope to convince you that it is after all possible to change the world. If one of these ideas excites you, then so much the better: feel free to take the ball and run with it. I also hope, though, to inspire you to come up with your own possibilities. My goal is to create a world in which all people are working together to constantly make the world a better place to live.

So here are seven of my ideas.

1. Start an organization to promote positive cultural change.

This organization would be different from all others existing today in that it:

- would have no religious affiliations;

- would have no political affiliations (neither Democrat nor Republican, neither conservative nor liberal);

- would have no political ambitions (would not become an independent party, nor endorse candidates);

- would be based on something larger than a single issue;

- would transcend national and ethnic boundaries.

The organization should be based on some simple, general goal: "to enhance the quality of life for all humans today and in the future," let's say. Its sole goal would be to improve our culture. It would provide a neutral ground for assessing cultural beliefs and attitudes, and for promoting positive ones. Such an organization would tap into a large and pent-up demand for addressing cultural issues. Many of our politicians' biggest issues today are ones that are, ironically, not political issues. Politicians talk about eroding family values, even though values are not things that can be legislated. They rail against the evils of Hollywood, even though government censorship is obviously an unacceptable solution. And they make abortion a central issue, even though this has become primarily a personal moral issue in our society today.

Politicians talk about all of these cultural issues because they are important to their constituencies – even though these issues do not have political solutions. At the same time, discussions on these issues are so deeply rooted in religious dogma that they only serve to make the divisions deeper, rather than helping to achieve consensus.

An organization that tackled cultural issues head-on, without any built-in religious bias, could achieve broad support and tremendous impact. Its first task could be to propose a modern moral equivalent to the Ten Commandments: perhaps the Seventeen Suggestions?

2. Publish a magazine titled *Work*.

Make it about work, and workers. This is such an obvious idea that I can explain this magazine's absence from our global media only by resorting to theories of mass hypnosis on a scale never before imagined. We have all sorts of magazines for owners and investors. We also have selections ad nauseam for and about management. About the only modern communications vehicle we have for and about workers is the *Dilbert* cartoon strip, and its phenomenal success should tell someone something.

In addition to pointing out the failures of bone-headed management theories, such a magazine could help restore some of the dignity lacking in modern work practices. *Work* could seriously represent the viewpoint of workers, which is genuinely missing from our modern culture, in all places except the corporate lunchroom, the area surrounding the water cooler, and the local bar.

The only real barrier I can see to such a project would be the natural resistance of managers and investors to launching such a venture, since such a publication would inevitably expose the weaknesses of both.

3. Create a new independent political party.

Call it the Progressives (unless such a name is already in use). Found it upon the idea that, although modern democratic forms of government have been uniquely successful in preventing the worst sorts of abuse of power, they have proven not very effective or efficient at coping with our growing social problems. Build the identity of the party on basic principles, rather than current issues. Identify those principles and clearly prioritize them.

Find a middle ground between the two extremes advocated by our major political parties in the US. The Democrats often try to solve problems by sinking more of our tax dollars into the Federal government. This approach tends to create bloated, inefficient and ineffective bureaucracies. The Republicans tend to react by stripping the US government of all authority, and relying more on the power of the states and the private sector. This approach leaves no one in charge to protect the average citizen from unbridled corporate greed. The public finds it hard to get excited about either extreme, because they have little faith in any of these groups. Unlike the politicians, voters instinctively know that our form of government is based on a careful balance of power, and not on a blind faith in any one sector.

The current impasse between our major political parties is created by the false idea that either the Federal government has to do it all, or local governments and the private sector have to do it all. There is a third alternative, which is more reasonable. This third possibility is that the private sector should do most of the work, but that our central government should be more creative about establishing the rules by which citizens and business have to operate, so as to benefit society as a whole. (See some of my following ideas for examples of what I mean.)

This approach will offend big business and big government, because it will force both sides to work differently, and to each acknowledge their own weaknesses. But it will be popular with the people, because it will challenge both powers to work for the common good.

4. Make it easier to operate employee-owned businesses.

These forms of business would tend to unite the interests of owners, management and labor, and help to balance the interests of all three parties. Our current legal system, however, makes such forms of ownership awkward. Instead, we should have new legislation that makes it easy for people to come together in such relationships.

5. Outlaw discrimination based purely on the size of a business.

Modern corporations are growing larger all the time, with bigger companies regularly swallowing up their smaller competitors. Big business, of course, would have us believe that this is a natural and healthy phenomenon, based on supposed efficiencies created by economies of scale.

Workers in these corporations, though, will tell you that such hugeness also has its price. Layers of management become so deep that the people at the top often issue edicts that make no sense at all to the people on the bottom, who are the ones most in touch with the day-to-day realities of the business. (See almost any series of *Dilbert* cartoons for examples.)

The truth is that business size is also influenced by many common forms of discrimination that favor corporate behemoths. Volume discounts are one example. These are sometimes justified by real savings, but are more often given simply because they are customary, and because suppliers cannot afford to refuse such discounts when they are demanded by their largest customers.

Other examples are the shelf space fees commonly charged by grocery chains. Suppliers must pay large fees up front just for the privilege of being stocked on these chains' shelves. Small suppliers cannot afford these costs, and so are squeezed out. In other words, retailers decide which products to offer their customers, not based on which ones cost less, or are more pleasing to consumers, but first and foremost on who can afford to pay for the privilege.

Such discrimination threatens the very principles of individual initiative and enterprise upon which the United States has been built. These huge, monolithic corporations reduce competition, stifle individual creativity, and reduce rewards for individual efforts. In an immortal society, we must rely more on people, and less on faceless corporations.

Our economy would be much more flexible, dynamic and enterprising if we were to pass laws that would make it illegal to practice such forms of corporate discrimination. This would even the playing field between large and small competitors, increasing competition and passing on real benefits to consumers, workers and investors.

6. Implement environmental impact taxes.

Such taxes would make companies responsible for the long-term environmental impacts caused by their products. You would think that this would only be common sense, yet the US has been slow to fully implement such practices. This sort of taxation would end the pointless arguments between those who favor unregulated business, and environmentalists who would outlaw practices they consider harmful. Taxation would allow businesses maximum flexibility, but would make them pay the real costs of environmental degradation.

For example, products that are not recyclable would be charged a tax that would help pay for the cost of landfills. The tax would vary depending on how long it would take their products to decompose in such conditions. Lumber companies would pay a tax that would allow trees to be replanted and managed over the life of the "crop," when they log on public property. Automakers would be subject to a progressive tax that would increase with the amount of emissions produced by their products.

7. Outlaw advertising as we know it.

I'm referring to the kind of advertising that is "pushed" at consumers, rather than being "pulled" by them on demand. I realize that this idea sounds radical, because modern capitalism has become almost totally dependent on this form of advertising.

The law would prohibit sending people commercial information that they have not, in some way, specifically asked for. In other words, no more junk mail (whether sent by paper or electronic media). No more unsolicited phone calls from people trying to sell you something. No more commercials in the middle of your television shows. No more magazines that have more ads than copy.

The truth about most advertising today is that it represents a huge waste of resources. Companies spend tremendous budgets on advertising, simply because it is necessary to gain access to the markets. Yet these ads contain little or no information useful to consumers, other than letting them know that a new product is available, and how it is being positioned in the market. Much advertising is totally ignored, since it is pushed at people who have not asked for it. This entire activity is socially productive only in that it employs vast numbers of people who would otherwise have to find more useful employment.

The knee-jerk reaction of most businesses would be that such a law would cripple them, making it impossible for them to reach potential buyers. The truth is that it would simply require society to create other forms of commercial communication.

Some of this is already happening naturally on the World Wide Web. Businesses make information about their products available on their Web sites, but consumers only see this information when they actively seek it out. The powerful search services that are available make such focused information retrieval possible. This is a new paradigm, that makes the consumer responsible for actively seeking out information, rather than passively waiting to have such information thrust upon him. Other forms of information dissemination would also emerge, perhaps produced by organizations such as Consumers Union, publishers of *Consumer Reports.*

Another major objection to this law would come from the media, since they have become heavily dependent on revenues from advertisers. They would simply have to adapt, finding more direct ways to fund their activities, and perhaps limiting these activities to more affordable levels.

In the US, of course, objections would be based on our Constitutional right to free speech. Yet our founding fathers certainly never meant to imply that people had no right to choose whom to listen to. By pushing out unsolicited commercial messages to consumers of other products, or to unsuspecting mail recipients, consumers are regularly deprived of this choice. Ultimately, though, this law might require a Constitutional amendment to thoroughly avoid this objection. Such an amendment would in no way limit our rights of free speech, but would provide a Constitutional basis for our rights to free listening.

The social benefits of such a law would be tremendous. First, it would help level the playing field between big and small companies, since hugely expensive advertising campaigns would no longer be necessary to market a product. Second, it would empower consumers to make more informed decisions (since hardly anyone can pretend that current ads, despite their immense cost, deliver much useful information). Third, it would conserve the countless resources now almost entirely wasted by advertising (whole forests would be saved by the reduction in size of newspapers alone).

Fourth, and possibly most importantly, elimination of current forms of advertising would tremendously improve our culture. The vast amounts of trash produced by the popular media, mostly as a means of collecting advertising dollars, would no longer have a viable funding source. This does not mean that worthwhile efforts would no longer be funded. It simply means that entertainment would not be churned out on media assembly lines, simply to satisfy demands for quantity, rather than quality.

With such a law, it would no longer be so easy for consumers to become "couch potatoes" – passive recipients of the mass media. Consumers would have to become more discriminating. Since media would become more expensive, consumers would have to make more conscious choices about their consumption. Perhaps they would even have to find other avenues of entertainment, such as talking to each other, or listening to live entertainment. Such a law would also mean that the creators would tend to really have something to say, rather than simply being paid to produce "product."

The long-term effects of such legislation are hard to predict in detail. Given sufficient consideration, though, it is hard to imagine how they would not be supremely beneficial. The effects would be so far-reaching that they would produce in effect a new form of capitalism. This may offend people who think that we have already arrived at the perfect rules for our economy. It should only seem natural, though, to those who believe in our continuing evolution towards higher and more efficient forms of social organization.

Making A Difference

You may think that some of the ideas I have just shared with you are totally loony. That's OK with me. My point has not been to sell you on each and every one of these suggestions. What I hope to have accomplished, though, is to show you that it is possible to come up with new ideas that will change the world, and quite possibly for the better.

You may think it difficult, if not impossible, to accomplish such changes. But if only one of these ideas appealed to you, then why shouldn't it appeal to others as well? And if it appeals to many, then why shouldn't we collectively be able to make it happen? Implementation of ideas like these may be difficult – but I bet that such work will be more fun than watching TV.

After all, once we've made the decision to stay here forever, we may as well make the world the way we want it.

Chapter 37

Next Steps

I HOPE THAT THIS BOOK HAS STIRRED YOU to feel a greater excitement for living. If you feel a real passion to live, then you may be wondering where to go from here with this newfound aliveness. Your options are infinite, and limited only by your own imagination and daring. Following are a few ideas to get you started.

1. Read more on the subject.

I can recommend *Together Forever: An Invitation to be Physically Immortal,* by Charles Paul Brown, Bernadeane Brown and James Russell Strole. See the order form at the back of this book for more information. Also see the "Recommended Reading" list at the back of this book for further recommendations.

2. Meet regularly with others who are interested in physical immortality.

Groups of 5–12 people work best. Meet once a week or so. Discuss this book, or other ideas and feelings you have about living forever. Be careful not to engage in debate, though. Concentrate on supporting and inspiring each person to live better than they ever have before. Focus on the feelings you want to create – aliveness, and a nurturing love and respect for one another – rather than the importance of particular ideas.

Be physical, as well as mental. Don't be afraid of your feelings. Don't be afraid to touch one another. And don't be afraid of silence – holding hands and looking in one another's eyes can be as powerful as talking (and much more powerful than talk that is produced just to fill an empty space).

Encourage each person to express their original feelings, rather than just reacting to someone else. Select a moderator for each meeting, and rotate this assignment each week. Appreciate each other's differences, rather than trying to set some single standard for "expressions" at these meetings. Don't be afraid to be shallow, as well as deep. Have a good time, express your heartfelt feelings, and get closer to these people than you ever thought possible.

3. Attend a lecture, workshop or seminar on the subject of physical immortality.

Check our web site or the ForeverNet newsletter for a calendar of upcoming events on the subject of physical immortality.

4. Join the Living Forever Network – ForeverNet, for short!

You will receive a regular newsletter that will help you take the three steps I've listed above. We'll tell you about other books that are available, including in-depth reviews. Our calendar of upcoming events will help you connect with speakers and workshop leaders on the subject of physical immortality. And we will help you network with others in your area who are interested in immortality, so you can support each other. See the order form at the back of this book for information on how to receive a free copy of the newsletter. Or check out our World Wide Web site at http://www.powersurgepub.com.

5. Buy another copy of this book and give it to a friend.

Spread the word!

6. Give to others what you want for yourself.

Treat each person you meet as a fellow immortal.

7. Try something new!

Notes

1. Dr. Marc Grossman and Rachel Cooper, *Magic Eye: The 3D Guide* (Kansas City: Andrews and McMeel, 1995), page 23.
2. William Blake, "Auguries of Innocence" (1805), line 1.
3. The Bible, Book of John, verse 14:12, King James Version.
4. Dylan Thomas, "Do Not Go Gentle Into That Good Night"
5. Deepak Chopra, *Ageless Body, Timeless Mind: The Quantum Alternative To Growing Old* (New York: Harmony Books, 1993), page 307.
6. Woody Allen, *Without Feathers* (New York: Random House, 1975), page 99, "Death (A Play)."
7. Benjamin Franklin, letter to Jean Baptiste Le Roy, 13 Nov 1789.
8. Leonard Hayflick, *How And Why We Age* (New York: Ballantine Books, 1994), page 189.
9. Leonard Hayflick, *How And Why We Age* (New York: Ballantine Books, 1994), page 215.
10. Robert E. Ricklefs and Caleb E. Finch, *Aging: A Natural History* (New York: Scientific American Library, 1995), page 2.
11. The Bible, Book of Job, verses 33:22–25, King James Version.
12. The Bible, Book of 1 Corinthians, verse 15:26, King James Version.
13. The Bible, Book of John, verses 8:51–53, King James Version.

14 The Bible, Book of John, verse 8:58, King James Version.
15 Deepak Chopra, quoting Shankara, *Ageless Body, Timeless Mind: The Quantum Alternative to Growing Old* (New York: Harmony Books, 1993), page 53.
16 Deepak Chopra, *Ageless Body, Timeless Mind: The Quantum Alternative to Growing Old* (New York: Harmony Books, 1993), page 167.
17 William Ernest Henley, *Echoes* (1888), No. 4, In Memoriam R. T. Hamilton Bruce ("Invictus"), stanza 4.
18 The Bible, Book of 1 Corinthians, verse 15:26, King James Version.
19 The Bible, Book of Job, verses 33:22–24, King James Version.
20 The Bible, Book of Psalms, verses 102:19–20, King James Version.
21 The Bible, Book of Hosea, verse 13:14, King James Version.
22 The Bible, Book of 1 Corinthians, verses 15:51–53, King James Version.
23 Leonard Hayflick, *How And Why We Age* (New York: Ballantine Books, 1994), page 341.
24 Cathy Perlmutter with Therese Walsh, "Think Yourself Healthy," *Prevention*, August 1996, page 74.
25 Cathy Perlmutter with Therese Walsh, "Think Yourself Healthy," *Prevention*, August 1996, page 71.
26 Paul Pearsall, *Super Joy: In Love With Living* (New York: Doubleday, 1988), page 84.
27 Herbert Benson, "Think Yourself Healthy," *Prevention*, August 1996, page 71.
28 Paul Pearsall, *Super Joy: In Love With Living* (New York: Doubleday, 1988), pages 83–84.
29 Amit Goswami, *The Self-Aware Universe* (New York: G. P. Putnam's Sons, 1993), page 39.
30 Amit Goswami, *The Self-Aware Universe* (New York: G. P. Putnam's Sons, 1993), page 73.

31 Amit Goswami, *The Self-Aware Universe* (New York: G. P. Putnam's Sons, 1993), page 40.
32 Amit Goswami, *The Self-Aware Universe* (New York: G. P. Putnam's Sons, 1993), page 103.
33 A.G. Cairns-Smith, *Seven Clues to the Origin of Live* (Cambridge: Cambridge University Press, 1985), page 3.
34 A.G. Cairns-Smith, *Seven Clues to the Origin of Live* (Cambridge: Cambridge University Press, 1985), page 1.
35 Alfred, Lord Tennyson, *In Memoriam* (1850), 56, stanza 4.
36 James E. Lovelock, *The Ages of Gaia*.
37 Carl Sagan and Ann Druyan, *Shadows of Forgotten Ancestors: A Search for Who We Are* (New York: Ballantine Books, 1992), paperback, page 277.
38 Carl Sagan and Ann Druyan, *Shadows of Forgotten Ancestors: A Search for Who We Are* (New York: Ballantine Books, 1992), paperback, page 277.
39 *The American Heritage Dictionary*, Third Edition, definition 1.a.
40 Marshall Herbert McLuhan, *The Medium is the Massage* (1967).
41 Patrick Henry, Speech in Virginia Convention, Richmond (March 23, 1775).
42 The Bible, Book of Deuteronomy, verses 5:7–21, King James Version.
43 Thomas Jefferson, *Declaration of Independence* (1776).
44 *The American Heritage ® Dictionary of the English Language*, Third Edition (Houghton Mifflin Company, 1994).
45 The Bible, Genesis, verses 1:22, King James Version.
46 Karl Marx, *Critique of the Hegelian Philosophy of Right* (1844), "Introduction."

Recommended Reading

Physical Immortality

Together Forever: An Invitation to be Physically Immortal
by Charles Paul Brown, Bernadeane Brown and James Russell Strole
   This is a groundbreaking book on the subject of physical immortality. First published in 1990, this exciting work offers wonderful insights into what it means to live an immortal life.

The Immortalist
by Alan Harrington
   A thought-provoking work on the possibilities offered by human physical immortality.

Physical Immortality: The Science of Everlasting Life
by Leonard Orr
   An entire book on the subject of physical immortality, by the man known as the "father of rebirthing."

Rebirthing in the New Age
by Leonard Orr and Sondra Ray
   This is one of the pioneering books of the rebirthing and New Age movements. The book provides a good introduction to the immortalist philosophy as taught by most rebirthers.

Rebirthing: The Science of Enjoying All of Your Life
by Jim Leonard and Phil Laut

Another introduction to rebirthing, including a section on immortalist philosophy.

Healing Into Immortality: A New Spiritual Medicine of Healing Stories and Imagery
by Gerald Epstein, MD

This is a brave book that draws upon Western spiritual traditions to create a framework for healing, and even for physical immortality. The book offers many imagery exercises for healing health problems, increasing your energy, and even for "resurrection." More than just a collection of techniques, though, this book presents a broad spiritual structure for living. This structure is rooted in Western traditions, rather than the Eastern ones that have served as the basis for the work of modern healers such as Deepak Chopra.

The Revelation: Our Crisis is a Birth
(The Book of Co-Creation)
by Barbara Marx Hubbard

The "Revelation" of this book's title refers, in its first sense, to the Christian Bible's book of the same name. In fact, the bulk of Barbara Marx Hubbard's book consists of the text of the biblical book, interspersed with commentary from Hubbard, not only in her own voice, but also in a "Higher Voice," or "Christ voice." This latter commentary was communicated by a "Presence" that Hubbard says was "both within me, and beyond me … my Self and yet far more than myself."

This book is a brave attempt to reinterpret the Bible in terms that offer humanity hope for a future here on earth. The author boldly portrays our human potential in radical terms that may not fit easily into any existing stream of thought, whether it be Christian, scientific or New Age. Hubbard's vision and call to action are exciting ones that deserve a wide readership.

Fiction Depicting Physical Immortality

Forever Man
by George Michael Greider
    Forever Man is a smart, literate thriller that probes the themes of death and immortality. The author takes a fresh approach to these subjects, and produces a book that is entertaining, wise and ultimately life-affirming.

The Forever Machine
by Mark Clifton and Frank Riley
    Clifton and Riley won a Hugo award for this work of science fiction, first published in 1956. The book is about a machine that can confer immortality on people by clearing them of their neuroses, suppressions and mistaken cultural programming. The catch is that it only works if people are open to it. Although written forty years ago, the book seems dated in only the most minor and superficial ways. It still offers remarkable insights into the nature of our culture, and some remarkably fresh ideas on possible paths to immortality.

Jitterbug Perfume
by Tom Robbins
    First published in 1984, *Jitterbug Perfume* is an enchanting tale about a group of people who have been alive for centuries. Written in Tom Robbins' inimitable style, and reflecting his unique concerns, this book offers refreshingly positive attitudes towards the possibility of living forever. A lot of fun to read, as well.

The Spring
by Clifford Irving
   A yarn about what might happen when an isolated community discovers a fountain of youth in its midst. An exciting and thought-provoking tale.

Anti-Aging

Ageless Body, Timeless Mind: The Quantum Alternative To Growing Old
by Deepak Chopra
   In this book, Chopra turns his considerable talents to the subjects of aging and longevity. The result is a skillful blend of science and philosophy, of physics and biology, of East and West, and of general principles and specific practices.

The New Nutrition: Medicine For The Millennium
by Dr. Michael Colgan
   The author is one of the world's leading experts on nutritional supplements. Director and founder of the Institute that bears his name, he has served as a consultant to vitamin manufacturers, professional athletes and Hollywood celebrities. He has written several previous books – on sports nutrition, cancer and supplementation – but this is his most accessible work for general readers.

The Anti-Aging Plan: Strategies and Recipes for Extending Your Healthy Years
by Roy L. Walford, MD, and Lisa Walford
   Advice on healthy living through caloric reduction, the only technique that has been scientifically proven to extend the lifespans of laboratory animals. Roy Walford is a leading expert on gerontology, and was a member of the *Biosphere 2* team. Lisa is Roy's daughter, and is a chef and yoga instructor.

Never "Old": The Ultimate Success Story
by Jesse Anson Dawn
Never "Old" is an entertaining, inspiring and illuminating book on the subject of physical rejuvenation. Those seeking carefully validated scientific information about aging and longevity should be forewarned to look elsewhere. Dawn's approach to the subject is mostly anecdotal, based on his own experience and inspiration. What Dawn does offer is a refreshing attitude towards living and aging.

Wellness

Why Zebras Don't Get Ulcers: A Guide to Stress, Stress-Related Diseases, and Coping
by Robert M. Sapolsky
The cover of this book features a whimsical illustration of a group of graceful, carefree zebras holding hoofs and dancing in a circle. The book itself lives up to the cover's promise. One could easily imagine that reading a book about stress and its negative effects on the human body could itself be a supremely stressful experience. Sapolsky, however, manages the difficult feat of making his subject not only approachable, but actually fun.

General Science

Shadows of Forgotten Ancestors: A Search for Who We Are
by Carl Sagan and Ann Druyan
This book takes on the really big questions, like "What does it mean to be human?", and comes up with some intriguing answers. Using information from biology, psychology and evolution, the authors shed intense illumination on their subject, and make it possible for readers to hold more informed

opinions, whatever their religious or philosophical predilections. A fascinating book of self-discovery for the human race, it ultimately made be proud to be human.

Index

- A -

abandonment 46, 94, 188
accidents 9, 29, 131, 132, 253, 267
Adams, Scott 64
afterlife 4, 19, 28, 34, 36, 59, 62,
  76, 77, 162, 171, 179, 215, 216,
  217, 218, 223, 224, 267, 268
Ageless Body, Timeless Mind
  36, 285, 286, 292
agelessness 102, 103, 212
aging 13, 20, 21, 32, 33, 37, 54, 61,
  65, 73, 89, 100 – 103,
  128 – 133, 174, 216, 285, 292,
  293
  reasons for 33
AIDS 79
alienation 94, 171
Allen, Woody 27, 28, 285
ancient secrets 22, 85
angels 19
apathy 188, 189
Arizona 7, 46, 107, 251
Armstrong, Neil 32
ascension 19, 62
Atlantis 19
attraction 105, 174, 187 – 194,
  196

- B -

Bambi 69
Bannister, Roger 22
Beatles, The 41

belief systems 52, 75, 78, 79, 113,
  152, 158, 212
BenDror, Raya 95
BenDror, Shmulik 95
Benson, Herbert 76, 286
Bible, The 34, 36, 57, 62, 221,
  253, 285 – 287, 290
  1 Corinthians 15:26 35, 58
  1 Corinthians 15:51–53 60
  Hosea 13:14 59
  Job 33:22–24 58
  Job 33:22–25 34
  John 14:12 23
  John 8:51–53 35
  John 8:58 35
  Psalms 102:19–20 59
biology 33, 125
Biosphere 2 107, 292
Blake, William xi, 285
bodywork 259
Bohr, Niels 123
Bonomie, Andres 95
Bowie, Pauline 45, 46, 95,
  251 – 256, 259
Bowie, Stephen 95, 253
breathing techniques 20, 45,
  259
brotherly love 187
Brown, Bernadeane v, 95, 251,
  281, 289
Brown, Charles Paul v, 95, 251,
  281, 289
bumper stickers 75
burial plots 86

businesses
  employee-owned 275
butterfly effect 121

– C –

cancer 5, 130, 292
capital punishment 159, 163
capitalism 141, 147 – 149, 186,
  187, 277, 280
Capra, Frank 43, 44
careers 5, 12, 44, 64, 66, 109, 132,
  133, 143, 170, 176, 243, 244,
  251
century plant 130
chaos 33, 109, 121, 123, 180
children 8 – 11, 66, 68, 80, 93,
  109, 129, 178, 185, 252 – 256
chimpanzee 135
Chopra, Deepak 27, 28, 36, 37,
  183, 199, 285, 286, 290, 292
Christ. See Jesus Christ
Christianity 22, 34, 36, 40, 57,
  62, 133, 221, 290, 291
co-creation 208, 236
Collard, Clem 95
Collard, Pat 95
college 8, 10, 42 – 44, 161
commandments 228
community vi, 12, 44, 46, 127,
  180, 214, 218, 222, 223, 228,
  292
competition 126 – 129, 133, 134,
  142, 143, 149, 151, 195, 196,
  235, 236, 276
computers 44, 137 – 141, 205
conservatives 196, 200
Constitution, US 170
corporations 64, 87, 136, 148,
  155, 195, 243, 275, 276

creativity 24, 95, 276
cult experts 170
cults 169, 170, 172
culture xii, 18, 43, 46, 69, 70, 71,
  139 – 142, 145, 147 – 150, 185,
  214, 235, 273, 274, 279, 291
  organization for positive
    change of 272
culture crisis 147, 148
cynicism 75

– D –

Darwin, Charles 91, 93, 126, 134,
  142, 241
death 27, 35
  acceptance of 29
  certainty of 31
  fear of 28
Death Becomes Her 20
death consciousness 180
Declaration of Independence
  244, 287
democracy 63, 87, 141, 186
desktop publishing 204, 205
determinism 120, 121, 200
devil 220. See also evil
Dilbert cartoon strip 64, 273,
  276
discrimination
  based on corporate size 275
diversity 41, 44, 46, 62, 134, 135,
  143
dominance 94, 136
Druyan, Ann 136, 287, 293

– E –

Easter Bunny 40
economic impacts 11

INDEX

economics 4, 147 – 149, 176, 177, 180, 181, 194, 195, 197, 276, 280
Eden, Garden of 133, 247, 260
Einstein, Albert 23, 24, 118, 177
elixirs 105
empowerment 53, 216, 220, 224
encounter weekends.
  See Gestalt therapy
endlessness 102
energy 6, 65, 117 – 119, 123, 125, 136, 179, 219, 231 – 234, 290
entrainment 199
entropy 119, 120, 220
environmental concerns 13, 68, 179, 181
evil 35, 91, 180, 214, 220, 222
evolution xiii, 91, 108, 112, 126 – 129, 134, 137, 139 – 143, 147 – 152, 167, 177, 196, 220, 241, 266, 280, 293
  cultural 91, 140, 141, 143, 147, 148, 152
  genetic 139 – 143, 177
exits to death 217
extraterrestrials 19

– F –

fables 20
family 9, 12, 39, 41 – 43, 45, 66, 67, 69, 80, 93, 106, 109, 129, 135, 136, 143, 145, 148, 160, 165, 166, 192, 195, 197, 252, 253, 255, 257, 273
feelings ix, xi, xii, 14, 16, 28, 30, 88, 92, 97, 98, 102, 108, 109, 160, 161, 165, 166, 171, 184, 187 – 189, 192, 193, 219, 222, 233, 236, 259, 282
Finch, Caleb E. 33, 285

flesh, human 34
flounder 130
Ford, Henry 64
foreverness ix, 98, 99, 102, 267, 269
fountain of youth 8, 85, 292
four-minute mile 22
Franklin, Benjamin 31, 285
free will 120

– G –

Gaia Hypothesis 135, 143
Galapagos tortoise 130
generation gap 178
genes 93, 129, 132, 135, 136, 139, 141, 145
gerontology 33, 61, 292
Gestalt therapy 44
God x, 14, 22, 36, 40, 48, 59, 67, 77, 90, 91, 102, 121, 158, 160, 162 – 164, 217, 218, 220 – 237, 241, 245, 261, 266
gorillas 135
government 11, 14, 63, 90, 91, 141, 169, 170, 187, 195, 197, 273 – 275
greater works 23
Greenbaum, Norman 171
group therapy.
  See Gestalt therapy

– H –

hardware 138, 139, 141, 142, 205
Hawking, Stephen 123
Hayflick, Leonard 33, 61, 285, 286
heaven xi, 19, 32, 34 – 36, 48, 59, 62, 163, 180, 194, 213 – 217, 221, 224, 267, 268

heaven on earth 32, 163, 215, 245, 247
Heisenberg, Werner 122
Heisenberg's uncertainty principle 121
hell 80, 180, 216, 247
Heller, Joseph 42
Hendrickson, Clendon 256
Henley, William Ernest 53, 286
higher power 72, 73, 76, 213, 214, 217, 218, 230, 245, 246
Holocaust 171
homosexuality 165
Honda Motor Company 64
human condition 42, 187, 215
human interaction,. *See* togetherness
humanism 245
hypertext 206, 207

– I –

Immortality Quotient xii, 52, 53, 71
incremental immortality 4
independence 226
individuality 41, 44, 92, 142, 143, 166, 235
insanity 47
insects 130, 142
insurance plans 65
interdependence 134, 143, 246
Internet 205 – 208
intimacy 188, 260, 261
intuition 233, 234
It Happened One Night 44
It's A Wonderful Life 44

– J –

Jefferson, Thomas 287

Jesus Christ 23, 35, 36, 187, 290
job. *See* careers

– K –

Koresh, David 170, 172
Kuhn, Thomas 23

– L –

liberals 196, 200
life 125
  quality of 32
life insurance 28, 86, 106
limitations
  absence of. *See* unlimited
Lion King, The 68
longevity 20
Lorenz, Edward 121
Lovelock, James E. 287
Loving Relationships Training 45
LRT. *See* Loving Relationships Training

– M –

magic 20
Magic Eye x, 285
martyrdom 159, 172
Marx, Karl 267, 287
Marxism 187
matter 117
McLuhan, Marshall 149
meaning of life 160
media, communications 28, 68, 109, 170, 187, 279
medicine, Western 183
Meet John Doe 44
morality 181, 222
Morris, Doug 236

Mr. Smith Goes to Washington 44
myths 20, 37, 100, 150

– N –

New Age thinking 36, 37, 45, 146, 212, 229, 230, 232, 289, 291
nourishment 94, 167, 188, 189, 260

– O –

On the Origin of Species 126
orangutans 135
Orr, Leonard 259, 289
outside the box thinking 25
overpopulation 9, 10, 13, 151, 163, 178, 181

– P –

paradigm shifts 23
parenting xiii, 66, 250, 251
patterns 121, 139, 144 – 146, 177, 234
Pearsall, Paul 76, 77, 286
People Connection. See togetherness
People Forever 46, 208, 251
perfection 37, 91, 160, 243, 267
physics 33, 112, 121, 123, 125, 232, 292
Pinerua, Veronica 95
political parties
 independent 274
pollution. See environmental concerns
Ponce de Leön 85
predation 131

Prevention magazine 72, 76, 286
primates 135, 136, 137, 139, 145, 232, 241
prosperity 242
psychology 6, 161, 293
purpose 160, 224, 245

– Q –

quality of life 8, 21, 65, 96, 151, 271, 272
quantum mechanics 122

– R –

Ray, Sondra 259, 289
Reagan, Ronald 163
rebirthing 45, 259, 260, 262, 289, 290
Reese, Jennifer 44
reincarnation 19, 36, 62, 215, 216
relationships 8, 16, 41, 43, 134, 166, 185, 186, 189, 204, 235, 261, 265, 275
relativity 23, 24
religion xiii, 4, 14, 28, 34, 37, 40, 42, 46, 58, 62, 76 – 78, 90, 113 – 115, 133, 148, 162, 166, 167, 170 – 172, 180, 192, 212 – 219, 221 – 225, 228, 229
 organized 227
reproduction 129, 130, 178
repulsion 186, 188, 189, 192, 196
responsibility 42, 46, 88, 89, 179, 214, 223, 224, 234 – 236, 265
retirement 10 – 12, 66, 67, 176
Ricklefs, Robert E. 33, 285
Right to Die movement 61, 70
royal jelly 130

– S –

sacred texts 14, 57, 222, 227
Sagan, Carl 136, 287, 293
salmon 130
Schrödinger, Erwin 122, 123
Schrödinger's cat 122 – 124
science 4, 23, 32, 34, 67, 68, 91,
   101, 107, 108, 111 – 115, 117,
   121, 123, 127, 135, 183, 184,
   192, 206, 218, 231, 232, 266,
   289 – 293
self-image 241
separation 37, 77, 81, 90, 94, 166,
   188, 222, 230, 234, 259 – 261,
   269
sexuality 165, 192, 252
Shadows of Forgotten Ancestors 287, 293
Shankara 37, 286
silver bullet 3, 85
Sisson, Colin 259
software 138 – 141, 205, 244
soul 34, 37, 53, 58, 135, 165, 166,
   209, 260, 261
space travel 32
spirit 37, 165, 166, 171, 214, 219,
   220, 230, 231
Spirit In The Sky 171
spirituality 14, 37, 261
Streep, Meryl 20
Strole, James Russell v, 95, 251,
   281, 289
Structure of Scientific Revolutions, The 23
submission 94, 136
suicide bombings 77
suicide, mass 171
Sukop, Egbert 95
Super Joy 286
Super Marital Sex 76
Superimmunity 76
synchronicity 233, 234

– T –

Teammate Appreciation Day 156
technology 147 – 149, 174, 186,
   203 – 209
television 4, 29, 44, 95, 147, 171,
   233, 277, 280
Ten Commandments 221, 273
Tennyson, Lord Alfred 287
terrorism 77
therapy, Gestalt. See Gestalt therapy
thermodynamics, second law of 33, 119, 120, 220
Thomas, Dylan 27, 29, 285
timelessness 99, 100, 102, 103
togetherness 14, 16, 39, 41, 44, 46,
   180, 184 – 186, 195, 196, 204,
   208, 222, 223, 226 – 228,
   235, 236
tower of Babel 77

– U –

uncertainty 48, 105, 121, 122
unconditional love 94
unity 226
universal laws 232
universe 22, 52, 73, 87, 92, 102,
   107, 108, 113, 117, 120, 123,
   136, 144, 164, 194, 200, 219,
   220, 232 – 234, 241, 242, 246
University of Michigan 42, 43
unknown 98, 106, 108, 109, 234
unlimited 73, 81, 102, 108, 176,
   231, 252, 262

– V –

values xiii, 87, 143, 148 – 150,
    153 – 160, 167, 172, 174, 214,
    221, 222, 224, 245, 273
victim consciousness 53, 55, 61,
    71, 132
violence 29, 59, 170, 180, 186, 188
virtual reality 203

– W –

Waco, Texas 154, 169 – 172
war 42, 94, 101, 159, 167
Watt, James 163
Weil, Andrew 183
wholeness 78, 96, 227, 228
wills 28, 86
word processors 138
workers
    magazine for 273
World Wide Web 206, 207, 278
Wright Brothers 22

– Y –

You Can't Take It With You 44
youthing 101

– Z –

Zemeckis, Robert 20

Order Form

If you would like to purchase additional copies of this book, please ask for it at your favorite bookstore. You may also order it directly from the publisher, using this form, or a reasonable reproduction thereof. You may also place your order using our toll-free number.

Title	Price	Qty.	Total
Why Die? A Beginner's Guide to Living Forever, by Herb Bowie (trade paperback)	12.95		
Together Forever: An Invitation to be Physically Immortal, by Charles Paul Brown, Bernadeane Brown and James Russell Strole (trade paperback)	9.95		
ForeverNet newsletter – Sample Copy	free!		free!
Postage and handling (per book)	2.95		
Total Amount			
Name:			
Address:			
City: State: Zip:			
Country: Telephone:			

Please make check payable to, and send order to:

PowerSurge
PUBLISHING

PO Box 14707
Scottsdale AZ 85267-4707 USA
1-602-451-6895
1-602-657-0727 Fax
1-800-925-3248 Orders
email: info@powersurgepub.com